PRAISE FOR
TRIATHLON FOR THE EVERY WOMAN

"This book is packed with useful insights that will not only support the reader's journey to an IRONMAN finish line, but also inspire and equip her to embrace endurance sport as a rewarding way of life."

   —ANDREW MESSICK, President and CEO, IRONMAN

"Women all over the world *can* do a triathlon. This book will show you how."

   —NICOLE DEBOOM, Founder of Skirt Sports

"This book is a must-read for every person who wants to change her life through my three favorite activities: swim, bike, run. Meredith's approach to triathlon training is both funny and detailed, effectively helping you reach your goal of crossing the finish line."

   —SENATOR KYRSTEN SINEMA (D-AZ), Chair,
   Women for Tri Advisory Committee

"You can become a triathlete. This book is proof that all you need is a little work, a lot of patience, and a spirit of never giving up."

   —DANI GRABOL, first female EPIC 5 Finisher and author

"*Triathlon for the Every Woman* tells the reader that she can do a triathlon in exactly as she is—in the space, place and body she has now. Meredith has proven that she doesn't let anything stand in her way—including herself. Now, she has readers believing this true gospel."

—LOUISE GREEN, author of *Big Fit Girl*

"Do yourself a favor and read this book multiple times. What will you learn? To simply work hard, believe in yourself, and just keep moving forward—that's all you need."

—MIRNA VALERIO, ultra-runner and
author of *A Beautiful Work in Progress*

"This book will start you on a journey of a lifetime. As Meredith says, 'Just Keep Moving Forward.'"

—JAMES LAWRENCE (The "Iron Cowboy"),
and author of *Redefine Impossible*

"Meredith Atwood and I are cut from the same cloth: we're both on a mission to help women get out of their own way. If you follow the tools as outlined in Meredith's book *Triathlon for the Every Woman*, you'll get the kick in the butt you need to bring your fitness (and your motivation!) to the next level."

—LAUREN HANDEL ZANDER, author of *Maybe It's You*,
Co-Founder and Chairwoman of Handel Group

"*Triathlon for the Every Woman* brings you up close and personal with Meredith's journey from couch to competition. Rich with useful tips for anyone contemplating a triathlon, the book is as much a metaphor for anyone who chooses to make a big decision to change her life."

—JOYCE SHULMAN, Founder and
Chief Macaroni Mom, Macaroni Kid

"This book will take you from wherever you are to the finish line of your first triathlon. You can be a triathlete—no matter who you are or what limitations might seem to exist. With the right spirit, attitude, will (or 'wheels'), you too can get to your goal finish line."

—BRENT PEASE, The Kyle Pease Foundation

"This book is an inspirational and practical guide for anyone who is ready to change her life through the sport of triathlon! Meredith, through her own personal journey, is proof that with a little sweat, determination, and a great sense of humor that you can change your life—and encourage other people to do the same."

—JACK SPARTZ, author of Moving the Middle

TRIATHLON
FOR THE
EVERY WOMAN

TRIATHLON
FOR THE
EVERY WOMAN

You Can Be a Triathlete. Yes. You.

Meredith Atwood

Da Capo

LIFE
LONG

Da Capo Press
Hachette Book Group
1290 Avenue of the Americas, New York, NY 10104
www.dacapopress.com
@DaCapoPress

Printed in the United States of America
First Da Capo Press Edition: March 2019
Published by Da Capo Press, an imprint of Perseus Books, LLC, a subsidiary of Hachette Book Group, Inc.

The Hachette Speakers Bureau provides a wide range of authors for speaking events. To find out more, go to www.hachettespeakersbureau.com or call (866) 376-6591.
The publisher is not responsible for websites (or their content) that are not owned by the publisher.

Print book interior design by Linda Mark.

Library of Congress Cataloging-in-Publication Data has been applied for.

ISBNs: 978-0-7382-8543-6 (paperback); 978-0-7382-8544-3 (ebook)

LSC-C

10 9 8 7 6 5 4 3 2 1

To Mombow.

I wish Every Woman could have had a grandmother like you.

I miss you. Every single day.

TRIATHLON

Tri·ath·lon—One of the best and most addicting forms of competition consisting of swimming, cycling, and running all at varying degrees of distances. Triathlon is not for the weak, for It puts the athlete in an indescribable amount of pain, but when the race is over, you want to do it again. **Anyone who downplays the difficulty of a triathlon or the classification of it as a sport should be beaten.**

—FROM URBAN DICTIONARY

CONTENTS

Contents

FOREWORD

EVERYTHING STARTS WITH A DECISION; PAGE 1 OF THIS BOOK IS no different—it's *precisely* where we join Meredith Atwood: with her Decision to become a triathlete. As Meredith shares her own real and heartfelt journey, going from the couch (and long hours at her law firm and new-momhood!) to triathlete, it's clear that her motive for sharing her story is to convince you that you can do it, too! This book is like talking to a friend who wants to share this really cool thing with you . . . and she isn't going to take no for an answer!

Nothing is sugar coated: the journey *will* be hard. There will be days when the self-doubt creeps in. There will be days when you can't do everything in your life—and half of it not even well—but you're reassured of two things: you can do hard stuff and it will be worth it. Gently your mind-set shifts from "I can't" to "I can and I will."

For the newbie triathlete, this book is a must-read! *Triathlon for the Every Woman* condenses what usually amounts to years of trial and error and hundreds of conversations with friends, acquaintances, coaches, and experts into one book. When I read it, I, too, was reminded of so many "aha!" moments I have had in the sport. (If only I read the chapter about protecting the Queen in year one of my triathlon-ing, I could have saved myself a lot of discomfort!)

Meredith has rallied her years of experience in the sport, as both a beginner, an athlete, and a coach, and along with friends and experts, shares this knowledge in manageable, relatable, and simple ways. The book is full of answers to the questions you don't want to ask—and addresses the things you haven't even thought about. Even seasoned tri-athletes will take something away from the training advice: who doesn't need a nudge to take recovery seriously or be reminded of the impor-tance of cleaning your bike!

The real magic of *Triathlon for the Every Woman* is how Meredith's experiences resonate with "the every" woman's experiences and strug-gles—both in life and in triathlon. You will chuckle companionably with her and at other times cry, "YES!"

Whoever you are and wherever you are in your triathlon journey, there is so much you can take from this book. Her message is simple: *just keep moving forward*. I believe in that wholeheartedly, too.

—Rachel Joyce
Professional triathlete,
IRONMAN *champion,* Mom

RACHEL JOYCE is a mom and an attorney turned professional triathlete. She is a five-time IRONMAN champion and two-time 70.3 champion and has finished runner-up twice at the IRONMAN World Championships in Kona, Hawaii. In 2017, Rachel returned to racing, having taken 2016 off to have her son, and went on to win two IRONMAN races less than a year after giving birth and in doing so qualified for the IRONMAN World Champion-ships for the eighth time. Outside of training and racing, Rachel is a passion-ate advocate for equality and increasing participation in sport by women, as well as a coach. **www.racheljoyce.org**

INTRODUCTION

I N THE HAZY MORNING OF AUGUST 2010, I WOKE UP AND DECIDED that I would become a triathlete.

My Decision was not particularly interesting, aside from the fact that I was superfat. And slow. And tired. And angry.

And of the three of the sports that make up triathlon (swimming, biking, and running), I had never done any real swimming, biking, or running. Well, I would sometimes run to Dairy Queen for a fantastically large treat with ice cream and M&Ms and . . . *never mind*. Okay, I would "run" to Dairy Queen. Pffft.

To add insult to injury, I was busy. Really busy. A mom of two kids under two years of age. Married. I worked full-time as a lawyer. I commuted twelve hours a week. But I was most busy being tired, fat, isolated, and angry.

In light of the stuff I had going on in my life, my Decision to become a triathlete felt insane. Where would I actually find the time? Even worse, the Decision was riddled with all sorts of odds against me, self-doubt, and sizing concerns. For years, I sat and wreaked havoc on myself by eating crap and drinking more crap. But with my Decision, I decided that I would not continue to destroy myself.

Did I have all the answers once I made my Decision? Not even close. But it *was* the beginning of a miraculous journey.

Little by little, I started moving forward. I walked. I ran. I cycled. I cried. I wore a bathing suit (*horror upon all holy horrors!*). I set goals. I chiseled away at workouts. I did some small races. I met people who believed in me. I met people who did *not* believe in me. But I started believing in myself, and I kept going.

And one year later, after kicking my own butt, I crossed the finish line at a half Ironman triathlon. IRONMAN 70.3 Miami was a race made up of 1.2 miles of swimming, followed by 56 miles of cycling, and topped off with a half marathon run of 13.1 miles. A total of 70.3 miles by water, two wheels, and foot. The race took me over seven hours to complete. I crossed the finish line wearing a size 10 running shoe and an XXL triathlon suit. I was probably the biggest girl within a 10-mile radius that day, but I was also huge in heart.

Since my Decision, I have finished dozens and dozens of triathlons and running races. The biggest crazy feat, however, came two years after IRONMAN 70.3 Miami, when I finished my first *full* IRONMAN in Coeur d'Alene, Idaho—a race consisting of 140.6 miles of insanity: 2.4 miles of swimming and 112 miles of cycling, topped off with a full marathon of 26.2 miles. I have since completed three more of these crazy races in Lake Placid, Louisville, and Wilmington, and a stand-alone marathon at Marine Corps Marathon as a wheelchair pusher with the Kyle Pease Foundation. Even stranger is that I keep racing and trying new aspects of swim, bike, and run—and beyond.

So. How in the world does someone like me go from a serious couch dweller to a bona fide triathlete—while juggling a life, a job, and a family?

This book is about showing you exactly *how* to do it. I will give you all the tools you need (and more than you may want!) to get to the finish line of your first (or perhaps, next) triathlon. I will share tons of information about swimming, biking, running, nutrition, mental strength, gear, and race day preparation. Not only that, but I've included some tips and humor about how to balance it all (life, kids, relationships) while keeping yourself happy and sane. If you are teetering on the triathlon edge—not knowing whether you really *want* to even give tri a try—I swear, this book will push you right on over!

This book is for the "Every Woman," which, yes, I realize is totally bad *grammatically*.

However, that's what makes the title funny—because who is anyone to define what "every" woman needs? We are all different, with different needs, bodies, and goals.

So, who is the Every Woman?

Well. She is me. She is you. She is young, middle-aged, old, tall, short, curvy, thin, average, single, married, partnered, divorced, widowed, with or without kids, with or without job, with or without animals, with or without money, with or without sanity.

I am the Every Woman who is overworked, overtired, and potentially underappreciated at any given moment. I am (still) chunky, covered in stretch marks, and hoarding a closet full of fancy jeans that I can't pull up past my thighs. I am the Every Woman who happens to also have a spouse, kids, bills, and laundry coming out of her ears. I am the Every Woman trying to be everything to everyone all the freaking time. I am trying to keep all the plates spinning without losing my ever-loving mind.

> I wrote this book because I do not want any woman to feel the way I felt back in 2010. Isolated. Sad. Angry.

And really, I am pretty sure I have just described most *every* woman I know. Well, I'm sure some readers aren't chunky or don't have stretch marks. (*You dirty wenches.*)

With so much going on, how in the heck does triathlon fit into your life? It *does*. I promise. I have experienced triathlon as a tired Every Woman, not as a superfit, well-rested, hottie mom. Not only that, but triathlon has made me unbelievably peaceful, happy, and (semi)sane. I have not stopped life or taken time off from working or hustling or the daily grind to make triathlon part of my reality. I also did not take time off to write this book. I just squeezed it in with the rest of the chaos. (I'm sure you'll find thousands of typos, but I was probably helping with homework at some point and forgot where I was.)

I wrote this book for two reasons.

First, no matter *who* you are or *where* you are in life, I believe you can experience the joy of becoming a triathlete. However, it's tough to know where to start. When I jumped into triathlon, I quickly realized that not a single resource available spoke to someone like me (the soon-to-be-locked-up-in-the-loony-bin Every Woman). No book or magazine could be purchased that told a real story of an Every Woman's journey from a stressed Mommy Dearest to a grounded Zen-master triathlete. (Unfortunately, I am not a grounded Zen-master, so we are still looking for *that* book). But I have lived the Every Woman experience of debt, struggles (and continuing struggles) with food and weight, addiction, stress, marriage, kids, terrible bosses, and an unfulfilling career—which I combined with a less-than-graceful swan dive into triathlon. So, I wrote *the* book I wish *I* had found years ago.

Second, so many people in my life have given me hope and inspiration while standing behind me, foot up my rear end, screaming, "Yes you can!" as loud and as long as I could tolerate. I owe these individuals so much. I owe them a thank-you, yes. But I owe them the duty of paying it forward, of sharing their life-changing core messages in the context of how they changed *me*. I have received e-mails and notes from the past few years, stating this book has been the jumping-off point for so many baby triathletes.

In summary, no matter how tired, chubby, lazy, or indifferent you may be right in this moment, today is a new day, full of new opportunities. Things can be better for you. And I think the sport of triathlon is one path to *better*.

Your road to becoming a triathlete starts out with a basic Decision.

It's simple. You just *decide* to become a triathlete. Sounds stupid? Sounds embarrassing? Sounds impossible? Perfect. You are right where you need to be. But it truly *is* simple:

You can float/doggie paddle/swim.

You can ride a tricycle/bicycle/tandem/hand-cycle.

You can walk/jog/run/wheel.

You can do all three back-to-back in a little race called a triathlon.

Even if you can't do any of it right now.

Even if you have disabilities and hurdles and major obstacles to overcome.

You can do this.

You *will* do this.

And that's all you need to decide. Make the Decision that you will.

You *will* move forward.

You *will* create your goals, and you *will* achieve.

Slowly but surely, you *will* do it.

Trust the process. Create your goals. Believe. And you will. Now, let's get started.

1 MAKING THE DECISION TO BECOME A TRIATHLETE

MAKING A DECISION TO CHANGE IS ALWAYS THE FIRST STEP TO actually changing. As such, the first step in my long list of brilliant advice about becoming a triathlete is to:

Decide to Become a Triathlete.
(No matter how you look on the outside.
No matter how badly you hurt on the inside.)

First, you might want to know more about triathlon in order to make an informed decision about whether you want to join the sporty cult of spandex-covered weirdos. You might have a few questions before you put on a hideous wetsuit and jump into a cold lake on a Sunday morning with a bunch of neoprene-clad freakazoids. You might want to know exactly how difficult those early-morning wake-up calls actually are—especially on days that feel more suitable for brunch than bloody foot blisters.

Alas, I am telling you too much already! I should not scare you away at this early juncture!

So, I am asking that you trust me. Trust me and believe that triathlon is something you *need* in your life, much like a washing machine. However, triathlon is also something that you *want* in your life. Like a partner who actually knows how to use the washing machine.

HOW THE DECISION HAPPENED TO ME

I was tired of life as it was. I was tired of me. I also considered a certain someone's comments about my ability to do a triathlon. This person looked me dead in the eyes and nonchalantly said:

"You could do a triathlon right now, if you really wanted to."

So, in August 2010, I made a simple, one-sentence Decision: *I have decided to become a triathlete.*

Notice that I did *not* say: I have decided to *do* a triathlon. Deciding to become a *triathlete* is different than completing a triathlon.

Deciding to *do* a triathlon is making a goal to complete a single event, to succeed in a solitary moment. You cross the finish line and you are done, and you can head for the Waffle House to celebrate.

Deciding to *become* a triathlete is a new game entirely. My Decision to become a triathlete indicated several things:

1. I intended to do more than just *one* triathlon.
2. I would identify myself with a group of people who were serious athletes.
3. I would learn about triathlon, including rules and safety, and the proper way to compete in a race.
4. I would *become* someone very strange to the outside, nontriathlon "real" world.
5. I would *become* someone NEW. I would change.

So, I decided exactly this. Then, I wrote it on the very first post of a blog: *I have decided to become a triathlete.* Then, I held my breath. And I felt a little sick at first. But interestingly, once I made that incredibly crazy, yet simple Decision—things began to change.

The Fat Stranger

During this time of my life, each day was freaking *Groundhog Day*: wake up, get ready for work, tend to two babies, and talk to (or argue with) the spouse. Each day, I would walk to the bathroom and look in the mirror. And every single day, there she was.

The Fat Stranger.

Who was this woman staring back at me? I had kinda gotten to know the Fat Stranger over the recent years. I would sometimes look in the mirror and ask the Fat Stranger questions like *How did this happen to you?* Sometimes, I would ask, *How did you let yourself get like this?* The Fat Stranger would just stare back, blankly, with absolutely no answers. She was a snobby bitch, that Fat Stranger.

I did not like her.

I did not appreciate the Fat Stranger's post-baby boobs or the jiggly butt that looked like it had been hit with Ping-Pong balls. I could find no beauty in the bags under the bloodshot green eyes. I saw no love in the flappy, bat-winged arms. I especially did not like the Fat Stranger's droopy belly. That belly, a saggy-skin house that had cultivated two babies, fourteen months apart. Didn't matter that she had actually grown *people* inside of her . . . I did not like *any part* of her.

The Fat Stranger was not a bad person. She was just someone I did not want to know (or see).

Then, I hated that I hated her. I wanted to love the Fat Stranger. I wanted to find self-love and accept her. I wanted to say, *It's okay that you feel like a shell of the person and athlete that you once were.* I wanted to hug her and say, *You'll be okay. Things will get better.* But the truth was, I didn't know whether that was true. I didn't like who she had become—inside or out.

So, instead of figuring out how to love her, I just hated her.

At the time of my Decision, I knew absolutely nothing about triathlon. I had no idea about swimming and biking and running. I was pretty sure that triathlon meant doing all three of those things in a row, but I was not sure in which order or how far.

I was very tender to the fact that I was completely out of shape, teetering on depressed and repulsive in my own eyes. Even when I told my parents about the blog and my Decision, they gave me a three-seconds-too-long pause before saying, "That's great, honey!" Their "that's great" did not have enough oomph behind it, and the pause? Well, it hurt. I looked for negativity from every place. When you look for it, you find it—it's everywhere. I was overly sensitive. I knew that. But I also hurt—everywhere. My insides (and my knees) literally hurt from so many different angles.

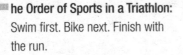

The Order of Sports in a Triathlon: Swim first. Bike next. Finish with the run.

But I had *decided*.

Something *had* to change.

And for once, I was going to stand by my Decision.

The Decision: The Turning Point

If you are *anything* like I was a few year ago, then you feel stressed, exhausted, and may have your own Fat Stranger staring you in the face. Or maybe she's a Sad Stranger. Or a Mad Mom. Doesn't matter *who*. But you may be staring back at someone you just don't like. I understand that.

When I started triathlon, I could border on saying I *hated* myself. That's gotten better over the years, but I still want to share these sentiments. And while reading about someone not liking herself can be a drag, I want to share the lows. I want to share the crazy inside my head, because I know that I am not alone—and I want you to know that, too (not that I am not alone. That *you* are not alone). I think it's important to speak the struggle, the self-loathing, the addictions and the issues that plague us . . . because so often that is very well our starting point. I thought I was alone; I was not. You might feel alone; you are not.

Adding another "thing" to your life may seem impossible. And piling on a preposterous statement like "I will become a triathlete" to the hectic mix may feel irresponsible and comical. (Lord knows, as women we cannot be irresponsible!)

Yes, the words are scary. The execution might be even scarier. But I am also convinced that those few words were the turning point of my life. Maybe I should repeat that. *Those few words were the turning point of my life.*

The. Turning. Point. Of. My. Life.

Becoming a triathlete required an epic shift in me, and the shift wasn't easy. And only a few months into training, I realized that I wanted many more things—not just in triathlon—but also in my life.

Becoming a triathlete is an amazing way to change your life and find *your* power. The Every Woman triathlon transformation is about more than simply looking better. Triathlon has the capability to transform your entire life. From your relationships to your job and your dreams. Will you look better? Maybe. A friendly side effect of triathlon is perhaps a better-looking body. But we are not talking about "30 Days to a Rocking Bikini Body."

Triathlon is not a gimmick that will take you to weight-loss nirvana. Triathlon is a bona fide sport. It's taken me over seven years to beat the "triathlon training to look better" ideal out of my subconscious. I do not think there is anything wrong with wanting to look better. But to talk, er, think, trash about my body, when it can swim, bike, and run for miles and miles? *That* is not only unhealthy—it's absurd.

Triathlon is a sport that works for working women with kids and significant others. It works for single women. It works for older women, smart women, funny women, silly women. It works for *women*. Triathlon works for women because there is so much spirit, love, and scheduling involved in swimming, biking, and running.

How? How will I find the time?

You will. And you will be surprised how triathlon becomes a part of your life. Just make your Decision to become a triathlete. The Decision does not have to be well informed. We women tend to make calculated, responsible, and well-informed decisions all the time. The Decision is not about making a well-thought-out-super-smart decision.

> Becoming a triathlete is an amazing way to change your life and find your power.

Seriously. Just make a completely blind leap with me. Decide to become a triathlete. The rest will follow. One step at a time, you will find a way. Cross my little heart.

WHO AM I TO TELL YOU . . . ANYTHING?

So, I made the Decision and I was instantly a triathlete! Ha. Okay. *No.* After making the Decision, I was a complete *flounder*, flopping all over the place, completely lost. I had made a bold statement, but I had no idea what to do next.

> "Tell me, what is it you plan to do with your one wild and precious life?"
> —MARY OLIVER

I ran a little. I flailed in the pool for a bit. I went to some indoor cycling classes. But after a few weeks, I was nowhere close to triathlon-ready. Really, I was just plain confused.

A Meredith History Lesson
1979

I was born a healthy baby, tipping the scales at a nice 8 pounds. My mom popped me out 100 percent naturally and drug-free, acting like it was no big deal.

1980–1987

I was a semifat kid. But I was one of those husky, strong specimens. "Give the bat to Meredith; she'll hit a home run," my dad would tell the softball coach. I would put down my doughnut on the bench and proceed to bat.

"She's strong!" everyone would say. But rarely did I hit the ball. However, I could punch the catcher in the face and then hit McDonald's for a tasty Filet-O-Fish if the situation called for it.

The truth of the matter: I really *was* strong. I was big and strong and I hated it. I picked on other kids because I felt like crap about myself. I was miserable and that misery caused me to eat more. I was lonely, so I ate. Then, I was fat and miserable, so I was mean. Food was my friend, my enemy.

1989

At age ten I started the Weight Watchers plan. Back in the late 1980s, no one knew that kids did not belong on a diet. My parents were faced with a portly kid, so they did the best they knew to do.

I entered the world of carrot sticks, cottage cheese, and water for lunch—also known as early-onset metabolic destruction. When I got home from school in the afternoon, I followed up lunch with secret handfuls of butter crackers. I stuffed those delicious round crackers in my cheeks so tight and so fast that my mouth would burst open and I would "poof" crumbs everywhere. I was just so hungry. My parents would go to sleep and I would creep to the kitchen for chips and cookies. My ten-year-old self would eat, eat, eat and then cry, cry, cry.

1990

I lost 10 pounds. I entered middle school weighing 125 pounds.

1991

By the time Aunt Flow arrived, I had shot up to 5 foot 7 and 155 pounds. Looking at pictures from that era, I was not obese. I played sports and was pretty healthy. But I believed I was fat, because I had *always* been fat. I was told I was fat. Fat was what I *knew*.

1997

I was a healthy teenager. I had a teenager pot belly, but overall I was fit and I worked hard at my sport of the time, Olympic weightlifting—competing at national and international levels.

("She's strong!" *Ugh*.)

But no matter how hard I worked, like many a seventeen-year-old girl, I spent entirely too much energy and time bemoaning my body, when hindsight shows me that I was actually kind of cute. Wasted cuteness. Wasted years and years of absolutely perfectly good cuteness.

In my wasted cuteness, I was still strong. I could hoist 220 pounds over my head and squat 300 pounds for sets. But really, all I could think about was my pot belly.

1998

I wore a pretty white dress to high school graduation. At the time, I thought I looked gross wearing it. Looking back, I was a babe.

New Year's Eve 1998

I began dating the Expert. Our first date was at Denny's—a 24-hour breakfast restaurant chain. A cup of coffee and romance at its finest.

Who is the Expert? That would be my husband, James. I lovingly refer to him as "the Expert" because simply put, the Expert knows *everything*, about everything. And if he doesn't, he will pretend he does. He's just a smarty-pants. He's also a good friend and an exceptional father. We've been together half of my life—so, life without him would be weird and empty. To the kids, there is no smarter man in the universe, so all is as it should be.

1999

I hung up the Olympic weightlifting belt and shoes.

Then, I started my second year of college in pursuit of the ever-useful English degree.

College was like college should be. I ate three pizzas a week, drank too much beer, and had more fun than you could shake a stick at. I also learned Latin, so I consider the college years a bloody smashing success.

2001

I graduated with a bachelor's degree from a Top 25 university. Time to make millions!

A few months later, the Expert put a ring on it and we were married. He was handsome and smart. I was a chubby, reasonably happy, twenty-one-year-old newlywed college graduate. *Hot dog.* I knew absolutely nothing about the real world, but I knew I was free to make my own decisions from that point forward. I liked that. Freedom was my new drink of choice. Freedom and bourbon.

2002

Newlywed-dom was awesome, and with my lucrative English degree, I made six dollars an hour selling discount eyeglasses in a college town. At night, the Expert and I drank beer and partied with our friends.

I have no idea what people complain about regarding the newlywed years. The Expert and I had awesome weekends without worrying about expectations, grades, or other foolishness. We had no real money, but we rented and ate on the cheap.

2002–2003

I decided that I could not bear to touch another moldy pair of eyeglasses and really, I *should* be doing *something* with my degree. Stupidly, I chose to go back to school to get another degree.

I got serious. Well, sort of serious. I watched every episode of *The Practice* on ABC. And I thought Dylan McDermott was a standard perk of any reasonable law firm. Henceforth and *ipso facto* and *res judicata*, law school seemed like a brilliant idea.

Unfortunately, three additional years of being glued to books by day and drinking beer by night did not do much for my health and waist. In my mind, I had absolutely no time for anything healthy. I had to *study*. All the time.

While other ladies in law school were picking out their fancy size 2 suits for interviews and running 5 miles before class, I was busting down the door of Cinnabon for a snack and then hitting the plus-size racks at the mall, begging the 22W relaxed pant to fit me so I could find a job, any job, any place.

During my third year of law school, the workload slowed, and I had a job lined up for my smashing future career as Ally "Only Fatter" McBeal. Because third year did not require the same intensity as the first two years, I was bored and had nothing to do but surf the Internet.

2004

In my loving new relationship with the World Wide Web, I found a nice mail-order prescription for a weight-loss drug. Apparently, you could just ask China to send you some and it would. I lost 50 pounds and entered Size Ten Land.

Along with my special pill, I had a specific meal plan to remain a resident of Size Ten Land. For breakfast, I ate an overprocessed low-calorie bagel with ultraprocessed low-fat cream cheese.

For lunch, I had Dog Food Soup. (Okay, so it was not actually dog food, but that's what The Expert called the pot roast soup I ate by the case. I can concede that it looked and smelled a tad like dog food. But it was 200 calories for the whole can. *Hot tamale!*)

I ate absolutely no snacks. I did not need snacks. I was not hungry, thanks to my phentermine addiction.

For dinner, I would eat a baked potato covered in fat-free shredded cheese, ketchup, and fat-free ranch dressing. I was stoked. I had found the miracle plan for skinny! I was finally skinny! It was so *simple*. Take speed pills, avoid alcohol, and eat severely limited quantities of beige foods. Genius!

I can now appreciate the fact that I was lucky to be *alive*, albeit in fabulous Size Ten Land, considering the havoc I was causing my body. I was very impressed with myself around this point in my life. I was "skinny." I was close to being a lawyer. I was headed for greatness, people! To me, skinny was obviously "healthy," so the next logical thing to do was *run*.

A few weeks after hitting Size Ten Land, I started regularly running miles on the treadmill, twice a week, at a fifteen-minute-mile pace. (In case you are wondering how fast that is—you can walk faster than that *right* now. Yes. Yes, you can.) The next logical thing? Enter a 5K (3.1-mile) race.

The Expert, who miraculously managed to avoid the fat plague until much later in our marriage, ran with me to encourage me. So, we ran, and completed the 5K in forty minutes.

2005

Two months after my first 5K, my father was involved in a near-fatal motorcycle accident, which sent our family into a tailspin. I started eating superbad brown food. I no longer cared about portion control. I also had no more money for my skinny pills. I was running on little to no sleep, hitting the road for a four-hour drive between home and law school several times a week.

My dad made it through and to my law school graduation. He was still in bad shape, but managed to make a fabulous hopped-up-on-oxycodone toast at my postgraduation party.

2005–2006

The Expert and I moved to a tiny little town. I took and passed the bar exam. We went to and hosted fabulous little parties. Gone were the "skinny" days. We spent weekends grilling out, partying with our neighbors, and lying about like slugs.

Size Ten Land became a vision in my rearview mirror, and my rear view grew wider. I flew right through Size Twelve Town, Size Fourteen City, and took up a seemingly permanent residence in the booming metropolis of Size Sixteen on a Good Day.

I loved our country house on 2 acres. I loved the quiet, the homemade guacamole, Sunday back porch sitting, and twelve packs of Coronas. The slow life—the turning-once-again ultra-unhealthy life.

I adored that town, but I hated practicing law there. (Turns out, I do not like practicing law anywhere, but that's neither here nor there.) When the stress with my boss grew, I ate more and drank more. I had loads of free time, but I learned to bake amazing cookies, instead of exercising.

2007

Of course, the perfect time to have a baby is when stress levels are high and you have absolutely no clue who *you* really are. I found out I was pregnant relatively quickly and things started to unravel at work. So I did what you did when you are pregnant and hate your job: I started looking. By the grace of God, a firm in Atlanta hired me *five months pregnant*. So, five months pregnant and with three weeks' notice, we put our country house on the market, packed up, and hauled our stuff to an overpriced apartment in a suburb of Atlanta.

> This was when the Fat Stranger made her debut appearance.

I had an easy pregnancy with our first child, James. However, the forty-plus-hour labor was the stuff of horror movies. The Expert and I left the hospital only twelve hours after James was born, because I wanted *out* of that hospital and *into* an Arby's roast beef sandwich and curly fries.

James was a cute baby who looked just a little like an old man with a side part. He was cranky like an old man, too. I was breastfeeding constantly. I was dog-tired. After three months of new mothering, feeding this strange old-man baby and waking up every two hours, I slogged my way back into the office, hauling my gargantuan breast pump and wearing stretchy pants. (Not that I minded the stretchy pants.)

In the *Groundhog Day* of the working stiffs, I woke up at five thirty each morning, pumped, dressed, and fought Atlanta traffic. I worked nine hours, ate lunch at my desk, pumped twice, spent hours and hours in traffic, and then picked James up from daycare.

I talked to the Fat Stranger on my commute into work. I would mumble things to her, stream-of-consciousness crazy, Faulkner-like: *This is not how I thought motherhood would be. Why does this kid cry all the time? How can I continue to work like this? I mean, how fat can I get before someone says something to me? Are the authorities going to commit me because I am ballooning up to the size of a whale? Would I be required to buy an extra airplane seat right now? Pitiful. I'm so gross . . . Ooooh! Snap. There's Dairy Queen . . .*

2008

One very special Cinco de Mayo Monday when James was barely six months old, I had yet another *Groundhog Day*. I was drenched in sweat by the time I picked up James from daycare. It was only eighty degrees outside, but I was 4,000 pounds. My feet hurt because I had spent the day in court, traipsing my heavy ass around downtown Atlanta in a too-tight suit paired with too-small heels.

On that day, the Expert was home early. And I will never forget the next moment as long as I live.

I was standing in the kitchen, eating butter crackers (flashback to my childhood) and watching James bopping around in his Exersaucer. My mind started to wander. *I wonder when Memorial Day is. Is it the nine-teenth or the twenty-sixth? If it's the twenty-sixth, then I think the Expert will be here and we'll go down to see my folks. That's only, what, two to three weeks? Like twenty days. Twenty days. Nineteen days? Nineteen days . . .*

I gasped.

I began counting. *Twenty-eight, twenty-nine, thirty, thirty-one, thirty-two.* That kind of *counting*. The ticking in the mind. *Thirty-three, thirty-four . . . days.* The pause.

I was late.

(Yes, *that* kind of late.)

I looked at baby James. He grinned a four-toothed grin at me. I looked at the Expert, typing away on his computer.

"I have to go to the store," I screamed suddenly, already halfway out the door. I pulled the door shut and almost fell down the stairs, I was trucking so fast. I drove the three blocks to Walgreens, hopped out of the car, and scurried down the aisles until I found what I was looking for.

Five minutes later—okay, that's a lie because I also went down the street and got a large strawberry milk shake with whipped cream . . . so, fifteen minutes later—I was back home. I locked myself in the bathroom with my milk shake and a First Response pregnancy test.

I looked at the Fat Stranger in the mirror and thought, *Oh, no no no no no no no no no.*

I peed on the stick. By the time the pee hit the indicator window: two pink lines. *Two pink lines. Two pink lines.*

I wandered out of the bathroom with the magic life-changing pee-stick in hand. Baby James started screaming from his post in the bouncy thing. *Time to feed the baby bird again,* I thought. The Expert glanced up from his computer. I waved the First Response in the air from across the room.

"What is that?" he asked. A glimmer of recognition flashed across his face.

"Oh," he said.

I nodded, tears welling up in my eyes.

"Oh?"

"Yes," I said.

"Oh. Oh!" His eyes roamed over to the screaming baby. "Oh."

"Yeah," I said.

New Year's Eve 2008

Once the shock wore off (four months later), I was excited to be welcoming a new member to Team Girl in the house. In celebration of Team Girl, I ate cheesecake almost every night.

Only fourteen months after James was born, I was experiencing déjà vu—sitting in the same labor and delivery room as I had with James. The Expert went off to find himself a sandwich, figuring the pony show would take as long as the last one.

Five seconds after the Expert left, the anesthesiologist arrived to give me the epidural.

Ooops. I was on my own.

"Hi, there. I'm Dr. John Malkovich" [okay, maybe that wasn't his name] "and I am here to give you the epidural. Please sit up and turn around," he said.

"How are you feeling?" he asked. I leaned back and looked at him. *What a doofus. Glad I am letting this joker stick a needle in my spine.*

"I'll let you take a guess," I said.

"Uhmmm, hmmmmm. Okay. What's your height and weight?" Dr. Malkovich asked.

I mumbled something.

"I'm sorry, didn't hear you," he said.

I mumbled again, "Five seven and a half."

"Okay," he said. "And your weight?"

I mumbled again.

"Ma'am, I need to know your weight—"

"Two eighty!" I screamed.

He jumped. Then looked at me for just a second in disbelief.

"Two hundred and eighty pounds," I whispered, embarrassed.

He eyed me carefully.

I started babbling, "Yes, I know, two hundred and eighty pounds is horrible. I know I know I know *I know!*" I squealed, "But the sooner you get this baby out of me, the sooner I will not weigh exactly that!"

A few hours later, out flew a feisty New Year's Eve baby girl, Stella, who still believes that all fireworks on December thirty-first are in her honor.

2009

Suddenly, these two incredibly small people, fourteen months apart and virtually helpless, were in our lives. All the time. I was shocked at how the kids never went away. Ever. There they were—every night and day. Cute and precious, and also bad and cranky.

The Expert and I trudged along. We moved out of our tiny apartment and began to fill a small house in a semi-icky neighborhood with kid stuffs: diapers, bottles, and squeaky toys. Topping the junk with full-time work, more breastfeeding, traffic, a new mortgage, sleep deprivation, and unbelievable amounts of squishy body parts was alarming. And stretch marks. *And what is* that—*a whisker?!* WTF.

When I returned to work after six weeks of maternity leave, I was a complete disaster. I was enormous, sleep-deprived, and angry. So angry. I constantly thought: *I am not a good mother. I can't handle this.* I felt absolutely hopeless. I did not know what to do or how to make myself feel better. Looking back, I think there is a real chance I had postpartum depression going on, but I did not care to figure it out at the time.

In a desperate attempt to find some sanity, I signed the Expert and myself up for a second 5K race. We had two months to prepare for it. He and I both tried to walk/jog/run over the next two months, but of course, there was no time. (However, we did find time to relax with wine and pizza and television when the kids were quiet.)

Despite the crappy training schedule, we still finished the race. I will not lie, however. The experience was humiliating and heartbreaking. I was heaving. My chest hurt. By noon, I was dizzy and nauseated. I physically felt terrible for two days.

I was not particularly hopeful about running or doing better after that race. I was unsure how to handle my feelings of hopelessness and stress. The day after the race, I had bruises on the bottoms of my feet from just those 3 miles.

I knew one thing: I really, really, really did not like the Fat Stranger. I did not like that she was unable to run. I was getting angrier and more hostile by the day. I hated the Fat Stranger to the point of tears and a Big Mac. I hated her even more when a co-worker returned from *her* maternity leave, looking like she'd had a tummy tuck and had been raising her newborn on a spa vacation.

I wanted to kill the Fat Stranger. Somehow. Without killing myself, of course.

Did Somebody Say Lunch?

On one particular morning, the baby monitor rattled with Stella's screams. She was eight months old. Shortly after, James (almost two) started wailing, too. The Expert was frustrated because he was heading out of town on business. I was frustrated because I had slept about three hours and I had forgotten to pick up my dry cleaning the day before. The dry cleaning that had my only size 20 suit. The one suit that actually fit me. The one freaking suit I needed for court that day.

I dug deep in the closet and found a hideous brown number with a supertight waist and a miserable high-water pant. The children did not poop or throw up on me before I left, so I considered that a win. As I drove toward the courthouse in downtown, I received an e-mail from my assistant on my BlackBerry: *Hearing postponed. Judge had family emergency.* Yes!

An hour later, I was at my desk with my breast pump shoved neatly in a drawer and my fingers flying fast and furiously across my computer keyboard. I felt okay, although my stomach was hurting from the tight pants. An e-mail hit my inbox at around nine o'clock:

> Lunch and Learn Session Today
> Noon
> Large Conference Room

Hot dog! Did somebody say lunch? Those lunches had the best box sandwiches with chips and cookies. I hit the Reply button and locked in my reservation for the meeting.

One minute before noon, I hovered outside the conference room, taking in the scent of the glorious cookies. Only then did I realize that the lunch session was presented by the gym located downstairs. *Great,* I muttered. *Gym membership sales. Super. Super. Super.*

I listened haphazardly and smacked on my sandwich thinking, *Yeah, these dumb people thinking I have time for this. When am I going to work out? When? When? When?*

"Five thirty a.m." said the leader, "The club opens at five thirty in the morning."

I snickered to myself. *And these gym memberships are always year-long contracts and I am not going to be stuck in . . . ,* but she read my mind again.

"The membership is month to month with a thirty-day cancellation policy."

Smartass fit lady, I thought, reaching for another cookie.

As I listened to the presentation, I thought, *Well, maybe I should join this gym. I could come to work a tad earlier, avoid traffic, and shower at the gym.*

Maybe.

By the end of the Lunch, I had Learned myself a sandwich, chips, three cookies, and a gym membership. I was a member. The sign-up included a free gym bag. *Bonus!* After the meeting, our firm's CFO walked over to me. "I am glad you joined the gym. I'm a member, too."

"Oh, yeah?" I said.

"It's a great gym. I could show you around sometime. You know, I could show you how to use the weights and the machines. Show you how to work out," he offered.

I stared at him. *Did he really just say that? I could "show you how to work out"?*

Then, I heard an explosion. Inside my head. *Boom!* I nodded numbly and turned away whispering, "Thanks."

I suppose that I appreciated the gesture. The CFO dude was simply trying to be nice, helpful. *How nice. How nice. How nice*, I repeated in my head in between head explosions. *Boom! How nice!* But I was incredibly humiliated.

And oh, was I mad! *I had once been an athlete, a weightlifter! I knew my way around a gym, especially the weights! Who did he think he was?*

I realized that my *past* athletic prowess was completely lost on others. The prowess was lost, because said prowess was actually invisible. I apparently looked as if I had never even heard of a gym, let alone had been a national-champion weightlifter. My feelings were hurt. I was mad at our CFO. But I realized, he was just stating the obvious.

I Showed Him

I stewed the rest of the afternoon at my desk and stewed during my miserable commute home. "I could show you how to work out." *Hurmph!*

I walked in the door to our apartment and stripped off my tight brown suit. I massaged my belly skin where the waistband had made a mark, cursed the Fat Stranger, and slid into my stretchy pants. James started screaming as I fed Stella. The house was a mess. The noise was epic. I was crying and stewing and battling the children. My ancient

BlackBerry was going *Ding! Ding! Ding!* Was I was living in an actual zoo?

Amid all the tangible chaos, all I could think about was the CFO offering to show me around the gym. *Dammit! Damn him! Damn all of this!* I was mad. Mad. Mad.

I was so mad that I dialed Pizza Hut.

An hour later, I had five pieces of stuffed crust pizza in my gullet, washed down with two (four?) beers. The Expert came home a little while later and finished off the rest.

"Hey," I said to the Expert after we put the kids down to bed and planted ourselves squarely in front of the television, "I joined a gym today."

He looked at me. Then, he looked back to the television. *Silence.*

"I got a free gym bag."

He would not look at me. He did not say anything. He didn't have to. I knew what he was thinking. Aside from his concern for the *cost* of the gym membership, he had utterly lost faith in my ability to do anything athletic. I never realized his disappointment in me until that particular moment. I saw it in his eyes. He did not mean to show it. His disappointment was not deliberate. It was not hateful. It just, well, was.

The Spark

The Expert and I did not speak the rest of the night.

I retreated to our bedroom, hurt and angry, but with a fresh beer. *This is my last beer ever*, I thought. I threw my brand-new gym bag on the bed. Slowly and muttering to myself, I dug through drawers, filled up little bags of toiletries, and packed for the gym the next day. I found an old water bottle. Finally, I tucked my shiny new gym membership card into the corner pocket of the bag, set my alarm, and fell into bed.

I woke up a little earlier than usual. The house was dark and quiet. By the light of the closet, I threw on clothes and sneakers, leaving the Expert and babies sleeping soundly. The traffic was nonexistent at that time of morning and I made it to the office in around twenty-five minutes, a significant improvement from the usual hour. Instead of plopping down at my desk, I dropped off my purse and headed downstairs to the gym.

It was September 11, 2009. I was petrified of the shiny new gym. I scanned my membership card and picked up a group fitness class schedule.

SPINNING® CLASS
Indoor Cycling

6:00 a.m.
Instructor: Gerry

I glanced at the clock above the membership desk. *Bingo.* I walked into the cycling studio about fifteen minutes early. The room was wrapped in mirrors and buzzing like Macy's on Black Friday. Music was playing over speakers, bikes were whirring. I spotted only one open bike near the back row and I snagged it. I fumbled with raising the seat on the bike, raising and lowering the handlebars. When I figured it out best I could, I sat on the bike and fitted my feet into the cages on the pedals. My rear end immediately hurt from the pressure of my weight. I was already out of breath as I began to pedal.

I finally looked around.

I was the largest person in the room by a good 60 pounds. I was also the most fashionable person in the room, wearing an extra-large gray T-shirt with some fat-lady leggings. My eyes scanned the mirrors.

Then I saw her.

The Fat Stranger.

Only this time I did not acknowledge *the Fat Stranger*. Instead, I looked into her eyes and chose to acknowledge the *person* who was really there. I acknowledged the sad and miserable woman.

Ugh. *Me.*

I turned my eyes away from the mirror, blinking and resolving to keep my eyes straight ahead for the remainder of the hour. The instructor was prepping his bike at the front of the class. I guessed he was the Gerry from the schedule.

I noticed a few things about this Gerry guy straightaway. He was ridiculously fit. And he was clearly a cyclist or a reality television star (or something equally as fabulous). Another thing about Gerry: he was very loud.

"Good morning," Gerry shouted. I looked up and braced myself.

Everyone shouted back, "Good morning!" I glanced around again. *This place is a freak show*, I thought. Most everyone in the class was fit, regardless of their age. *Fit fit fit*. I was an outsider. I was *not fit not fit not fit*. Gerry looked directly at me. I guess I stood out. Going forward, I avoided eye contact at all costs.

From the front of the class, he congratulated someone who had apparently just finished an IRONMAN. Everyone clapped. *Ironman? The movie?*

He gave a quick overview of the plan for the class and punched a button for the music. I stared at his spandex shorts and thought, *Those are very tight pants. Only a man in that kind of shape could wear something so ridiculous and still look amazing.*

"Close your eyes," Gerry said. I snapped back to reality from the boom of his voice, my legs beginning to burn from the few moments I had been pedaling.

"Think about what you want to accomplish today," he said. "Leave everything else outside. For the next hour, be here. Be here now. Be grateful."

The music was loud. I was grateful for that. No one could hear me huffing and puffing. I loved the song blaring through the speakers. I was in a crowd of freakishly ripped people, but I felt an intense loneliness. I was so lonely, so sad that I could taste it.

After the prior night with the Expert, the shame of my unfitness, the weariness of being a new mother twice over, the hatred of my job, I was left with nothing but disappointment in myself. Tears filled up my field of vision and rolled down my cheeks. I wiped furiously at my eyes, but the weeping continued. I could see my reflection in the mirror out of the corner of my eye. Hot, scrunchy-cry-face was happening. I was embarrassed for crying, but I was more embarrassed at the person I had become. Not just physically, although my body played a large role in the comedy theater of my situation.

But I was embarrassed for the *whole* person I had become. Angry. Huge. Isolated.

Be here. Be grateful.

I struggled with the pedals. I continued to move my legs, cycling through three or four songs and huffing profusely. Gerry shouted motivational words across the room. The music resounded loudly, until one song line hit me in the gut. I had heard the song a few times before, but had never given the lyrics much thought. In the cycling studio, it seemed that I was hearing them for the first time. The lyrics said something about every day, and the first day, and the rest of your life.

The tears came again. My exhaustion, my stretch marks, and my ferocious hatred for the Fat Stranger were washed away. All of the serendipitous moments of the prior two days had culminated in Gerry's cycling class.

In place of the anger, I felt a *spark*.

Yes, it sounds like total cheeseball-flimflam, but I felt a spark inside my core, a comforting warmth and then a fire of sorts. For the first time, I understood that every day was *literally* a new day and the first day of the *rest* of my life. That small understanding changed something inside of me.

Sure, all my responsibilities fell back on me when I walked out of the gym. But during that one hour in *that* class, I was *somewhere* else. I was *someone* else. *Was cycling class always that freeing? Would I be able to escape and figure out who I was if I came more often? Would more exercise give me that peace? Was this really something special? Was it a double rainbow? What did it all meeeean???*

On that day, I met the Fat Stranger with open eyes and a grateful heart, and I decided I would begin to like her. (Or at the very least, learn to get along with her, and figure out who she was.)

Early 2010

I continued to go to Gerry's class off and on. I loved the class, but I did not change a single bad habit. I went to the gym to run sometimes, too. The Fat Stranger and I became friends, all right. My standard week's schedule looked like this:

> **Friday**—Early-morning cycling class. Bagel with egg for breakfast. Eat nothing else all day. Mexican, margaritas, beer, and cheese-covered-deliciousness for dinner. Followed by ice cream and handfuls of Goldfish crackers until bedtime.
>
> **Saturday**—Recover from Friday night's fun. Take kids to breakfast. Eat greasy meal to soak up the alcohol. Take kids to ridiculous all-day outing like the zoo or aquarium, then eat greasy lunch. Ice cream. Put kids down for a nap. Dinner, wine, and more ice cream.
>
> **Sunday**—Recover from Saturday night's fun. Similar to Saturday except add "clean the frat house" and "wash all the clothes." Most important, declare Monday as the day to get in shape and eat well.
>
> **Monday**—Go to gym early in the morning, eat cookies by noon, and declare Mondays too stressful to make any real, calculated life changes. Drink wine at dinner (and after dinner) to tolerate the return to work on Tuesday.
>
> **Tuesday–Thursday**—Wake up ass-crack of dawn, get dressed, deal with kids, fight traffic, fight clients, fight my urge to murder everyone in the legal profession, fight traffic home, fight toddlers throughout dinner, sometimes fight with husband, and then drink wine to wind down, eat ice cream/Reese's cups and drink more wine, in order to stomach doing it all again the next day.

(Why was I so tired? I did not understand.)

I was still in an endless rut, even with my magical love for Spinning class. I was now friends with the Fat Stranger, but I was a little too friendly with her. Instead of just making friends with her, I was making *peace* with her. I was letting the Fat Stranger run my life, and give me all sorts of bad ideas and excuses.

The E-mail: Summer 2010

The kids were asleep. The Expert and I were chilling on the back deck with a couple of Heinekens. As I cracked open my fourth beer, I said to the Expert, "I don't know why I am so unhappy."

"Yeah," he said, "I don't know why, either."

The Expert is a lot of things, but unhappy has never been one of them. He's definitely the Tigger to my Eeyore.

"Maybe you should figure out why you are unhappy," he said.

"Yes, I would like to do that," I said. "And I have a sneaking suspicion that it has to do with me being an out-of-shape slug. And this beer."

"But the beer is delicious," he said, smiling.

"Yes, but this gut is not," I said, grabbing my overflowing belly.

"What about that cycling instructor guy?" the Expert asked.

"Gerry?" I asked. "What about him?"

"Didn't you say he was some sort of coach or trainer? You should ask him to help you," the Expert said.

"Really? He's really fit and looks busy and I think that—" I protested.

"Do you want to change or not?"

Looking back, that was THE question: *Do you want to change—or not?*

I thought for a moment. The Expert was right. After five beers, I found some bravery. I sent The E-mail to Gerry, asking for help. Help with my fitness. Help with my excess *me*. Help for a change. Just plain help.

The next morning, I woke up to find an e-mail in response. Because I had five beers, I guess I had forgotten that I had sent it. I was mildly horrified. But the damage had been done. I had declared an emergency state of change.

Gerry congratulated me on my desire to change and agreed to talk with me after class on Friday. I was nervous, wondering whether I had done something incredibly stupid.

I CAN DO A TRIATHLON! WAIT. RIGHT NOW?

I arrived to Spinning class early; Gerry made eye contact with me and waved. I had never talked to him before, even though I had been rolling into his class for almost a year. He must have figured out *who I was* based on the fact that I was the only me-size chick in his class. As we talked, he explained that he coached triathletes.

"Are you interested in triathlon?" he asked me.

He was standing very close to me and it made me super nervous. I was thinking, *Look, you crazy cute close-talker triathlete man, please take a step back or I am going to pass out from nervousness, high cholesterol, and your general badassery.*

He looked at me, waiting for a response (or proof of life).

"Um. Huh," I stuttered, completely confused. I didn't see that coming. I knew what triathlon was. At least, I thought I knew what it was. But I did not know what to say.

So, I said, "I hadn't really thought about triathlon."

"You could do a sprint triathlon. Right now. If you wanted to," Gerry said.

I must've stared at him as if he had three heads.

"You could!" he said. "I see how hard you work in class. You *could*."

I left our first meeting feeling a tad deflated. Not because of anything Gerry said, but because deep down in my gut, I knew I'd be flailing again before the end of the day.

Funny story, though. Less than seven weeks after my conversation with Gerry, I decided to make a run at triathlon. And that's when I made the Decision.

Gerry believed in me, and I started to believe in myself.

And . . . ?

So, why did I just tell you my entire life story?

Well, I believe that all women share similar struggles. For example, I have many beautiful friends with a banging hot body. I would kill to live in their body, just for an hour or even ten minutes (I would take off all my clothes and run through my old law firm buck naked during those ten minutes, too). It pains me to stand by and watch those women pinch their nonexistent belly and groan, *Ugh, look at this fat!* Also, it's not as though *fat* is the bloody worst thing to happen to us as people. For the love. It's *just* fat. But our culture makes it so much more—and therefore, so do we.

Regardless of your size and place in life, I am willing to bet that you might be living in the skin of your own Fat Stranger or Unhappy Person. Maybe you run through Size Two Land, but you are miserable for a myriad of other reasons.

I tell you about my timeline so you can see where I have been and how far I have come, simply by incorporating triathlon into my life and continuing to change and grow as the time passed. I hope that my story will encourage you and make you believe that you can do the same.

I was living my life as a Fat Stranger and made the Decision to become a triathlete. It was a crazy decision, but I knew that I was on to something. What exactly, I was unsure. I had so much to learn about triathlon. I set a goal, but I had no idea what to do next. I was a wannabe triathlete with absolutely no races scheduled and no plan.

I had no real resources. But I did have many questions. Questions, questions, and more questions. For instance: *What did I want out of the triathlon experience? What did being a triathlete really mean? How much and how often should I swim and bike and run? What is a transition? How far is a triathlon?*

Because I had no idea of the answers to any of these questions, I figured the quickest way to get to a triathlon was to sign up for a race. Almost immediately, the planning aspect of triathlon resonated with me. Professional triathletes pick their races sometimes years in advance. Most human beings need a schedule and a plan, whether they realize it or not. Moms of zillions of kids rely on the whiteboard calendar. As an attorney, my calendar was my lifeline and safeguard against malpractice.

I was excited when I could put triathlon on the calendar. I could search online for races, calendar the race, color code it, count it down, Facebook it, Tweet it, and iWhatever it. Yes. I liked it.

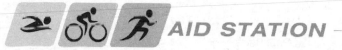 **AID STATION**

TYPES OF TRIATHLONS

The following table shows types and *approximate* distances of triathlon events. Individual races may vary slightly in distance, but the distance for each race is, more or less, as follows:

Type	Swim Distance	Bike Distance	Run Distance
Indoor Triathlon	200+ meters pool	30 minutes stationary bike	20–30 minutes treadmill
Super Sprint	Pool/lake swim	Short road bike	Short road run
Sprint	500–900 meters	10–18ish miles	3.1 miles (5K)
Olympic/ International Short Course	0.9 miles	25 miles	6.2 miles (10K)
70.3 Half Ironman	1.2 miles	56 miles	13.1 miles Half Marathon
ITU/Long Distance	2.5 miles (4K)	74 miles (120K)	18.6 miles (30K)
140.6 Ironman	2.4 miles	112 miles	26.2 miles Marathon

THE THREE TIERS OF GOALS

Gerry also suggested that I start making some triathlon race goals, and that I do so by *staggering* the goals and creating tiers of ambition.

The tiered approach is basically a three-part triathlon goal management system. Because research has clearly revealed that people like things in threes (swim, bike, run—peanut butter, jelly, bread—Moe, Larry, Curly—chips, salsa, cheese dip), the three-tiered goal system is harmonious.

For the purpose of the Every Woman triathlon journey, the Three Tiers of Goals are:

Quick Goal Race	1–3 months
Main Goal Race	6–12 months
Crazy Goal Race	2–25+ years

The Quick Goal is a race goal with a two- or three-month turnaround. You will want to have several Quick Goals during the year, to keep you moving and shaking. These might be known as the "B" or "C" races.

The Main Goal is the big deal race of the year—also known as the "A" Race in the triathlon world. This is your big race, the semiscary goal. Ideally, this would be the end of the season or end of year finale. The Main Goal is the thing that motivates you in your training. When people ask you what you are training for, the Main Goal is the race you shout out.

Finally, the Crazy Goal is just that. *Cuh-ray-zee*. Absolutely huge, mind-boggling, and seemingly never-gonna-happen.

The Quick Goal: 2–3 Month Plan

With the Quick Goal, you are setting yourself up for a quick win. The Quick Goal is a reasonable goal that, with a little steady work, you can easily attain in two or three months. Three months is an eternity in the fitness world. Trust me on this! You will be absolutely amazed to see the progress you can make in twelve weeks *if* you are diligent.

The point of the Quick Goal? Pure and simple, two things: Confidence booster! Habit former! By setting this goal and working toward it, you will get into the habit of working out and form a good trajectory for your future. Then, when you complete the goal, you will feel great and want to continue! You are setting yourself up for big things in the future, but you schedule these happy Quick Goals to boost your mojo.

So, what should you plan for your Quick Goal? Ask yourself some questions and evaluate your current fitness state. For a person new to fitness, a 5K running race is a great place to start. If you were to walk 3.1 miles, it would take you close to an hour to complete. If you jog it, maybe forty minutes.

My mantra and trademark is "Just keep moving forward." That's because forward is the jam! Forward is the pace to go. Forward is a pace.

AID STATION

RUNNING DISTANCE CONVERSIONS

Kilometers/Type	Miles
5k	3.1
10k	6.2
20k	12.4
Half Marathon	13.1
Marathon	26.2

You need not choose a running event for your quick goal—it can truly be anything fitness-related that gets you moving.

Here are some questions to ask when you are planning for the Quick Goal, in the case of a running event:

- Can I walk for 15 minutes now?
- Can I jog a mile?
- Can I walk 3 miles?
- Can I jog 3 miles?
- Would any of those things kill me?

- How long has it been since I've exercised?
- How long will it conceivably take me to run/walk/jog 3 miles if I work at it, with a plan in place?
- If someone threatened my life ("Run this far, or else!"), how far could I run right now, today?

For the last one, if someone walked into my house stating, "I will kill you *all* right now unless you put on your shoes and run ten miles without stopping"—then I believe I would run 10 miles without stopping. I cannot say the same about 38 miles. I would definitely *try*, but I absolutely do not believe I could run 38 miles without stopping. Right now? *No way. My poor dead family. Poor dead me.*

I honestly believe that *anyone* can run/walk a 5K within twelve weeks. So what if you can only walk for five minutes right now? Well, you can walk for eight minutes next week. And twelve minutes the next week, and so forth.

The 5K distance is absolutely doable for your first race, no matter who you are. I will repeat: *No matter who you are.*

Now, you may not be able to *run* the entire race, but you can certainly walk it and more than likely, you will run-jog-walk it. You can certainly move forward one step at a time and cross the finish line. If you plan well, you might be able to run the whole thing for your very first race. If you have never in your life run a 5K, then *who cares* whether you walk the race? Who cares whether you jog it very slowly? How you "run" your race is *up to you*. Don't forget it. This is your journey. These goals are *your goals* and you must not ever compare your goals to anything other than those ambitions in your head. Also, please note that when I use the word *run*, I am using it for simplicity's sake. I am very slow. I barely jog. I say *run* because *swim bike jog* doesn't have the same ring as *swim bike run*.

You may be coming to the table with some running experience already. My advice to you is to use the home-invasion analogy and schedule that distance race for two to three months out.

I made my Decision and I planned for a 5K about ten weeks later. Then, I registered for it. I finished it. And the rest is history. (Or something like that.)

My First Quick Goal: 5K

On the first Saturday in October 2010, I left the house before the sun came up. I was nervous. I only had a few goals etched in stone: (1) run the entire race; and (2) finish in less than forty minutes. The first half mile of the race was a steady incline, followed shortly thereafter by another quarter-mile incline. I was sucking serious wind right from the start. My heart pounded in my chest and I was breathing heavily. My legs were lead and everything hurt. But I jogged the entire race and my pace came in faster than I had hoped.

Quick Goal #1: Check!

Not only was crossing that finish line a victory, but it was symbolic. My race number was 2010. As I crossed under the FINISH banner, I looked down at my race number.

2010. The year everything changed.

My Second (Way Too Quick) Quick Goal

I tend to do most things a little too quickly. In deciding to become a triathlete, I fully intended to take time to become acclimated to triathlon things—to go slowly, to learn.

But my first Quick Goal felt amazing! I wanted more! I began to look for the next month's goal. *Maybe I could do a sprint triathlon! Maybe!* I searched online. It was October. I learned that triathlon has a "season" that is pretty much over in October. I would be forced to wait until spring to do an actual triathlon.

Humph. I could do another 5K, I thought. *That would be practical.* But something haunted me. I was scared. I was scared that the Fat Stranger would get comfortable in the winter sweaters, eating the Christmas cookies, and I might lose momentum.

Then, I saw it.

October tenth. 10/10/10. The last triathlon of the Georgia season. Appropriately named "The Last Chance Triathlon." I had only actually ridden my bike *three* times since the Decision. I had been Spinning many times. I swam a few times. But my thinking was: *Last Chance! Now or never!* Not my smartest move, but I had seven days to get ready for my first triathlon. Yes, seven days.

(Do as I say, not as I do.)

A couple of things about jumping into my first triathlon so quickly: first, it *was* way too soon. I *did* injure myself, and I am still plagued with a form of that original injury, years later. I also had had a pretty humiliating (yet exhilarating) race. However, to say I was "bit by the triathlon bug" would be an understatement. I was eaten *alive* by the triathlon bug after that race. And I would not trade it for the world.

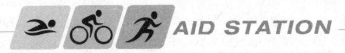

AID STATION

MY FIRST TRIATHLON

My first tri was a mere month after my big Decision to become a triathlete. It was, luckily, a sprint distance *reverse* triathlon: run, bike, and then finish with a swim.

My goal was to finish. That was it.

I arrived about an hour before race start. It was October and cold. I had completely forgotten a jacket. That stupid oversight made me wonder what else I forgot. I had a checklist, but this was my first time at the show. I wandered to the registration desk, picked up my number, and someone wrote all over me with a permanent marker.

I hauled my stuff over to transition and found a place to park the bike. Unlike at some races, there were no assigned spaces for the bikes. I laid out my gear. I put my bike on the rack. *Nope, wrong way.* I flipped it around. *Okay.*

The race announcer gave us the rules and a summary of the course. Before I knew it, the race started, and I was jogging. Remember this was a reverse triathlon, so the runners took off and they were zooooooming.

continues

continued

I finished the trail run, passing about six walkers, with my 5K time around thirty-eight minutes.

The transition from run to bike was pretty fast and smooth and flawless for the big klutz. I even clipped into my pedals without incident. I gulped down a strawberry gel during the first mile on the bike. My first gel ever. *Wow. Just as horrible as I imagined.*

My bike-handling skills were terrible. I was terrified the entire time on the bike. Corners, manholes, and cracks in the road completely unraveled me. At Mile 2.5, a massive hill appeared out of nowhere. I was heaving and puffing like a 400-pound smoker. This was really my first ride in the hills. Ever. I was sucking wind hard enough that people in *front* of me heard me coming, looked *behind* at me, and glared, perhaps thinking a train was on their heels. I watched as other riders acknowledged the horribleness of the hill and one by one, dismounted their bike and began walking up the hill.

I was suffering in the smallest gear, squeaking like rusty wheels, but I was *not* getting off that bike. My body was screaming, *WTF Stooooop!*

But I refused.

Around Mile 4, that evil hill was done. However, the course consisted of one hill after another. Still, I found myself finishing the 12 miles with very little drama, but with a very sore rear end. Plus, I seriously was terrified. I realized that I had not ridden my bike nearly enough to be out on a race course. I could not wait to get off the bike.

As I biked into the crowded transition area, I noticed a large spectator crowd. I saw one of the race volunteers pointing at me and waving his arms. He was screaming, "Dismount your bike! Dismount here! Dismount! *Dismount!*"

I panicked. I clipped my right foot out of the pedal, but my left foot was stuck. I braked hard and tried to avoid hitting the volunteer. I did not hit him. But I hit the pavement and hit hard, landing on the same left hip that began to throb during the run.

Those few seconds happened in slow motion. Me hitting the pavement. My jiggling body reverberating for ten seconds after the hit. The crowd gasping, followed by "Ooooooh!" When I stood up, they let out a big "Ahhhhhh" of relief and clapped.

continues

continued

The same volunteer who scared me with his "dismount! dismount!" shenanigans had rushed over after the fall and tried to pick me up under my armpits like I was a toddler. He was about 120 pounds.

"No, no, no no no no no no; I've got it," I said, when I really wanted to scream, *If you try and pick me up, Small Fry, I am SO going to bring you down to the ground with me.*

I felt like a clown. The sports photographer continued to take pictures of me. *Really, dude? Really?* I ignored him, because I still had a swim to do. I unbuckled and unlatched everything and ran to the pool.

Another volunteer was screaming, "No diving! No diving!"

No diving? *Uh, I have that under control.* I forgot my swim cap in transition, so my hair was flopping in my face, but the pool swim was a piece of cake. Before I knew it, a preteen helped wrench me out of the pool (I tried not to unintentionally take *him* down with me), and I was finished.

I totally overdid myself with my first tri. I rushed into it and I was hurting after the race—big time. Regardless, I was elated.

After all, I had finished my first tri! But then, just as quickly as I was thrilled, I had the nerve to ponder whether the race had made me an actual triathlete. However, I seriously hesitated to use the word *athlete* . . . let alone *triathlete*.

Was I a triathlete? I doubted it.

But that was stupid. I had just done a *triathlon*. It was time to figure out what was next, to keep going. So, I began to seriously think about what was next.

Triathlon is a massive learning process. I am *not* advocating jumping into a first triathlon as hurriedly and as stupidly as I did. Take your time. That said, I *am* advocating stepping out and embracing the fear factor(s) you may have. Because really, the fear is the worst aspect of jumping into something new. The brain between your ears will be your absolutely biggest—and worst—asset during this journey. Do not let your mind bully your body.

The Main Goal: The One Year-ish Plan

After an initial Quick Goal or Goals, you are ready to set your Main Goal. The Main Goal can be anything in the world, but it should be something that a home invasion could *not* make happen today. The Main Goal is something to complete in six months to a year.

Yes, the Every Woman journey is about making bold moves and strong decisions, but that does not necessarily mean rushing into goals either. I *will*, however, advocate the importance of reaching outside *your* comfort zone in creating your Main Goal. You must s-t-r-e-t-c-h to grasp something worthwhile.

If your goal is to become a triathlete, but you are very new to fitness, then your Main Goal could be a sprint triathlon. If, for example, you had only ever run a 5K and had never swam nor biked, then setting a goal for a sprint triathlon nine months down the road would be a very (very!) attainable goal. Or maybe running a 10K and focusing on a single sport, such as continuing with running, is easier to digest before tackling a triathlon.

Up to you! This is *your* path! What would *you* like to achieve? No matter the Main Goal, the goal should be something feasible for you to accomplish in six months to a year.

In creating your Main Goal, you should also put your money where your *mind* is. If you set the Main Goal, then register for it. Pay your money, mark the calendar, and tell someone.

Be Kind to Yourself

I can promise you a few things: You *will* fall down. You *will* struggle. You *will* question whether the triathlon decision is worth it. Others *will* make fun of you. They might say cruel things to you. Do not forget that you are experiencing a process. Do not give up on yourself.

During this progression, you will be learning about a sport, but you will also be learning about *yourself*. You may not like the person you have been for many years. You may be filled with regret. Strangely, triathlon will help you work through these emotions because you will be experiencing yourself in a new way. No matter where you start and where you go, remember four words: Be. Kind. To. Yourself. Your journey will lead you to the person you want to be; perhaps the person you were *meant* to be.

On the path to the Main Goal, continue to set up new Quick Goals every month or so. These can be on your training plan or in small races. Again, this is about setting up and experiencing the small wins and obtaining small successes. You will naturally see your 5K races feel stronger, get faster, and become more fun instead of frightening. These Quick Goals will help build your sense of control, strength, determination, and success.

> Remember to take care of yourself and *treat yourself gently* as you begin.

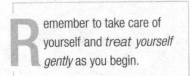 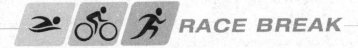 **RACE BREAK**

MY FIRST OFFICIAL "MAIN GOAL"

Soon after that first tri, I registered for St. Anthony's Triathlon—a classic race consisting of a 0.9-mile swim, 24-mile bike, and 10K (6.2-mile) run. I had five months to get ready. St. Anthony's was my first experience with a big-time race registration.

I called to tell the Expert. He said, "Awesome!"

I laughed.

"Well, hold your horses," I said before he hung up.

"What?"

"I am registering you, too."

He was silent. I heard a sound (a gulp? a sigh?).

"Sounds like fun," he said quietly.

The Crazy Goal: The 2–25 Year Plan

The Crazy Goal is something mind-boggling—something that you cannot imagine in your wildest dreams completing.

You can set Quick Goals, but they should be *reasonable*. You can set ballsy goals (the Main Goal), but they should also be reasonable (even if scary) and eventually, home-invasion attainable. Likewise, the Crazy Goal is something that you have a hard time imagining—something that if you finished, you would expect someone to film a documentary about you. *But* because of the nature of the Crazy Goal, it is automatically a *long-term goal*. Not a quickie.

From the get-go with my triathlon goal-setting, I thought of IRON-MAN as my Crazy Goal. 140.6 miles of pure movement, crossing the finish and hoping the epic "Voice of IRONMAN," Mike Reilly, would say: "Meredith Atwood, you are absolutely insane, but you are also an IRONMAN!" At the time, this Crazy Goal seemed so very impossible, but I still thought about it. I set it. And then I slowly worked toward it.

I became an IRONMAN in 2013 in Coeur d'Alene, Idaho. And then I did the same distance race again in 2014. And was called out as IRON-MAN two more times in 2015. And then on my podcast in 2018, Mike Reilly gave me an additional personal, "Meredith Atwood, YOU are an IRONMAN," for just the hell of it.

So, as you can see, before you realize it, the Crazy Goal becomes closer to being possible—and then becomes exactly that: *possible*.

This is precisely the point of the Quick, Main, and Crazy. Once the crazy becomes sane, you are ready for even more crazy. You will be consistently moving forward, toward something bigger and better, while never blowing the bigger dreams by impossible expectations. As long as you remain focused on the Quick Goals, with an eye toward the Main Goal (obviously increasing or changing your Main Goals each "season" or year), the Crazy Goal creeps closer.

Corner of Quick and Main: Shout from the Rooftops

I walked into a job interview two months before my first Olympic distance race. I told the managing partner of the firm that if I were to be hired, I would need a few days off for a race.

"What kind of race?" he asked.

"Oh," I said, "you know, just a triathlon."

"Oh, that's good," he said. "Are you doing a sprint?"

"Well, actually it's an Olympic distance."

An ever-so slight pause. "Wow. How far is that?"

"Well, about one-mile swim, twenty-six on the bike, and then a 10K run."

A bigger pause and a strange nod. "Well, that's good." Pause. "Er, good luck."

I can hear you now: *Uh, so, you want me to tell someone?!*

Yes, I am sorry, but I do.

Tell someone who will be supportive of your goals, if possible. Obviously, we all have different circumstances and people in our lives. Some of us have supportive spouses, friends, and family. Others have buttheads for family members who beat them up emotionally at every turn. If you have no one in your life who will support your new quest, then *your* resolve must be strong from the outset.

(If you are unsure whether you can withstand hurtful comments or stares from others, then I understand if you need to keep your goals quiet until you are certain you have become strong enough to tolerate the negativity. You may be starting this voyage from a place of rawness, a place resulting from years of sadness or defeat.)

Be prepared for the doubtful looks, the questioning eyes from others around you. I do not think it is necessarily malice, but oftentimes the looks are more . . . confusion. Terror. Curiosity. Disbelief.

At the time you set your Goals, you may not look like you can walk to the car without falling down. That's fine. Do not tell people that you have "decided to become a triathlete," which will certainly result in some nutzo stares. But telling others about your *race plans* is important. Once the phrase "I have a race that weekend" leaves your lips, you will feel things begin to change.

Keep the Crazy to Yourself

As far as the Crazy Goal is concerned, write it on a piece of paper and slip it into your sock drawer where you will see it sometimes. Tape it to the bathroom mirror. Make it your phone screensaver. But don't tell others about the Crazy Goal (unless they, too, are crazy). Once you begin triathlon, everyone outside of the sport will already think you are a loon. Leave well enough alone. The Crazy should stay in your head (for now) or be shared only with the small group of fellow triathlon crazies that you will later meet.

2 GETTING STARTED

I MADE THE DECISION! I SET THE GOALS! WHAT THE F AM I GOING to do now? I did what any English major–lawyer would do: I began reading and reading and reading about triathlon. I accumulated a few books for beginner triathletes, books about sprint triathlons, and checklists for necessary gear. I picked up a copy of Jayne Williams's book *Slow Fat Triathlete*[1] (henceforth known as *SFT*). Oh, *SFT* was a fire starter. The tagline for that book is "Living your athletic dreams in the body you have now." She obviously wrote that book just for me. (Just as I wrote *this* book for you.)

I had been holding on to this ideal: *If I lose weight, then I can run. If I lose weight, then I can do a race. Then maybe I will wear cute clothes to the gym.* *SFT* basically said to forget that ideal. Become who you want to be *now*. In the body you have *now*. That was life-changing for me, and I adopted it wholeheartedly. So, I pass that little wisdom on to you: *What are you waiting for? Be who you want to be now! Go go go!*

I am a bit of a type A personality. The *SFT* philosophy was a little more relaxed than I am capable of, even on Valium. (Not that I'm on Valium.) For starters, I believe in whole body, soul, family, and job *immersion* into triathlon. Not like a cult. But a wholehearted, healthy immersion—a schedule and a goal-setting plan that becomes a big part of your everyday life. Incorporating triathlon into the threads of your life is a vital component to successes in triathlon *and* life, no matter how small those successes may be.

I also believe that changing your body (or wanting to change your body) is *not* a bad thing. I believe that you should get moving *right now*, but I also see no harm in wanting to wear a bikini or desiring to have a six-pack under your shirt. I also believe that you must celebrate the body you have now, not for the way it *looks*—but for the awesome things it can *do*. Triathlon can bring that to your life.

For some people, having triathlon as a weekend fun "hobby" is enough. You may be okay with a few races here and there—and that is super. Every little bit of dedication and inspiration is life-changing. But I swear, for the true Every Women of the world, triathlon becomes a *necessary* schedule and foundation for a hectic day-to-day life. The immersion method is healing, methodical, and cathartic. You will want to kill far fewer people in your daily life if you buy into the sport—hook, line, and sinker.

Triathlon also walks hand in hand with your spiritual foundation, if you have one or desire one. You will talk to your God more than you ever have before. *Dear God, make this run stop. Dear Lord, I swear I will never eat again if you can just make this hill climb end. Heavenly Father, please take away my bicycle so I no longer put myself through this pain. God, please let the pool be closed today . . .*

So, while I will often draw on the *SFT* ideal of tri-ing in the body I have now, the Every Woman philosophy is a whole-life method—a little more extreme. The Every Woman way takes into account the partner, friend, mother, daughter, employee, etc., balance that triathlon will make better. Be who you *are*, most definitely—but strive to be the best *you* possible. Move forward in the body you have now, yes. But dream bigger than the outside world can imagine or understand.

Start in the body you are living in right now. Do it for *you*. And no one else. Then, go a step farther. Set the Crazy Goals—and, that's right, lady—dream big.

THE GREAT GYM CAPER

You need a gym to do this triathlon thing, I'm afraid. If not, then you need the outdoors or a treadmill, a bike or a bike trainer, and a lake or lap pool at your estate.

Get a Gym Membership with a Pool

You will need a pool if you are thinking of triathlon (ah-hem, *swim*, bike, and run). So, get a gym with a pool. The ole YMCA usually has a pool (bonus: with lifeguards) and a very reasonable membership plan. Sometimes, if you have friends join you, they may have reciprocal discounts.

The Mega Gym

A Mega Gym is one of those giant chain gyms, such as Life Time, Bally's, or LA Fitness. If you live near and can afford the Mega Gym, go forth and be a Mega Gym member! I promise you won't be sorry.

First, the Mega Gym will have a large pool with lap lanes. Waiting on a lap lane for swimming may remain a necessary evil, but the Mega Gym lanes rotate more quickly. With the resources and staff to tend to pool maintenance, the Mega Gym is less likely to have the infamous "Pool Closed for Cleaning" sign propped up for weeks on end.

Additionally, the Mega Gym will often have swim equipment, such as kick boards and pull floats, readily available. This doesn't seem like a big deal until you are juggling high heels, a suit and a wet pull float under your arm on your way to work. I speak from experience. Dry suit + wet pull float = ridiculous morning.

The Mega Gym will have numerous group fitness classes, lots of open-door time (often 24 hours) and state-of-the-art equipment. It will usually have multiple locations, so you access all locations with your one membership wherever they may be located. (If you are a traveling employee, this is the shizzle. And, um, no real excuse to skip a workout. "Oh, I just can't get to the gym today." *Wrong* (insert buzzer sound here).)

Finally, the Mega Gym will usually have childcare (a.k.a. babysitters!). This small factor will become priceless (if you have kids). The fact that someone at your gym will play with your kidlets while you catch an hour-long swim and quick run is 100 percent worth the extra coin. The kids will be exposed to fun activities and get in the habit of seeing Mom swim, bike, and run.

Worried about how expensive a membership might be? Well, you will be surprised by how much money you save not ordering Pizza Hut. It will easily pay for your gym membership(s). One large delivery pizza ordered every Friday night = $15 x 4 = $60 a month, plus tip. That's the difference between the YMCA and the Mega Gym . . . for your entire family. If you eat out more than once a week, start running those numbers and you'll have the money for your new road bike.

Just saying.

The 24-Hour Discount Gym

I love the 24-hour fitness places (e.g., Anytime Fitness or 24-Hour Fitness). Membership tends to be cheap. But usually those gyms don't have pools. If you can find a pool for free somewhere else (neighborhood pool, etc.), then the 24-hour gyms sans pool are a good option.

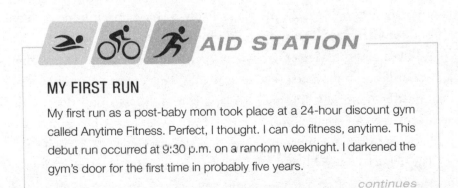

AID STATION

MY FIRST RUN

My first run as a post-baby mom took place at a 24-hour discount gym called Anytime Fitness. Perfect, I thought. I can do fitness, anytime. This debut run occurred at 9:30 p.m. on a random weeknight. I darkened the gym's door for the first time in probably five years.

continues

continued

Quiet. Ah. Peace and quiet.

I was wearing my old sneakers. The place was empty. I eyed the treadmill. I turned it on and started moving.

The workout was over almost before it began. I ran for *four minutes*, slogging around my post–baby weight, jiggling all over creation. *Four minutes*. I was at a 3.7 pace on the treadmill. Four minutes. And I was sucking wind as though someone had tried to suffocate me and I had finally succeeded in knocking them away.

The next day? Well, I could not move. I could not carry my baby girl up the stairs without crying because I had bruises on the bottoms of my feet. *Who cannot run for four minutes?!* I remember saying into the mirror with tears. *Who?!* The answer was: *Me. This girl. This girl can't run for four minutes.*

But I knew I could keep going. I knew I must. I knew I could do *fitness anytime*. Somehow, I did. I kept going.

Get a Membership to a Gym Near Where You Work

Really. By your office, job, fabulous place of employment is where you should make your gym home. If you are a working stay-at-home mom, then a gym near your house may be easier because your job *is* at home. See how easy?

Here's why: being a busy woman may require you to squeeze in workouts before the sane people (or your children or significant others) are awake.

In a nutshell, in the morning, you will wake up, head straight to the gym, work out, shower, snack, and have a short five- to ten-minute commute to your job, thus beating any traffic. If you obtain a gym membership by your house, it's easier to make an excuse to avoid it. *Oh, I woke up late. My commute is already behind schedule. Oh, I can sleep in if I skip.* It may not be statistically proven, but I've done both. Having the gym near the office is, hands down, the better route for triathlon. Plus, if you are lucky (and this is the best part), some days in the hot summer, you can sneak to the pool on your lunch break. No, not for your swim. But to take a mental health lunch and eat your food by the pool.

You might only be able to work out after work, for reasons related to schedules, family, or daycare. I urge you, however, to do your best to make morning workouts part of your routine . . . if at *all* possible. If not, then try to squeeze in your workout *immediately* after work—before going home and starting dinner and the kids' homework. If you can, hit the gym or the track directly on your way home from work—before the tornado of home responsibilities sucks you up. The later in the day you wait to train, the more likely the excuses will mysteriously appear.

If you have a long-ass commute, then you may need to explore a two-gym option. I'm not kidding, because you'll need your "home" gym on the weekends and your "work" gym during the week.

A Gym? But I Still Don't Have the Money.

I can appreciate that times are tough. But again, *this is about changing your life*. Women will sacrifice for children. Women will sacrifice for husbands. Women will sacrifice for church, pets, co-workers, and random people on the street. Now it's time for *you* to sacrifice . . . for *you*.

If the gym costs $80 a month, then clip coupons to save that amount of money in groceries. Turn off your cable. Figure it out, make a way. Push your sofa against the wall and get (steal, if necessary) a stationary bike and treadmill. Watch YouTube videos for crazy at-home workouts.

Simply put, there are *ways*. Most Every Woman *is* tired, money-tight, and out of shape. The question is: how much are you willing to give up? How much are you willing to sacrifice to have a better life?

ALL THE GEAR

If you are a gear and gadget junkie, then you have landed on a great sport. Three sports mean three times the paraphernalia, which equates to twelve times the confusion. You will need to budget for the *stuff* and figure out where to buy the *stuff*. Here's the quick and dirty scoop on the equipment needed to head toward your Main Goal as quickly as humanly possible.

First, a Few More Things

Budget: The stuff can get spendy, but it doesn't have to be. I make suggestions here for on-the-cheap options. Do not forget about searching online sales websites and groups. Or, just ask around. You never know who wants to get rid of a bike or wetsuit, yes, for *free*. Additionally, races will often have swim caps, water bottles, and discounted gear at the day-before-race expo events.

No budget: If you have and want to sink some cashola into a "hobby," you have chosen the right money pit. You will be surprised how quickly you will justify the extravagant expenditures for the sake of health, when really, you just want the shiny new Shimano shoes and Pearl Izumi arm warmers (in the summer). But I justify blowing cash for the benefit of my triathlon lifestyle because . . . *well, it's for my health.*

Repeat after me: *These fancy new socks are for my health. My $170 bike saddle is for my health.* Which actually, it is. A good saddle will save the Queen's health. (If you don't know who the Queen is yet, you will—especially if you skimp on a good saddle.)

Triathlon clothing and anyone over a size 0: You will learn that triathlon clothing can be exceptionally undersized, which can be incredibly discouraging for us normal to larger women. Thankfully, larger-size tri clothing exists now (it didn't when I started out), but be prepared to hunt for it (the power of Google) or to even wear men's sizes. Triathlon clothing is a market that is extremely oversaturated now—you can find practically anything for anyone—even in larger sizes.

Winter gear: I have not listed the essential winter gear you may need to run or ride outside. This list assumes that you will do most of your training indoors during the cold months, and hoping that you can catch the end-of-season winter sales for the next year.

Swim Gear

Swim clothing: *Swimsuit? Swimsuit? The horror!* Trust me, I completely understand. Still, if we are talking triathlon, we've gotta talk swimsuits.

The bad news: you cannot swim in a tankini with a skirt or board shorts. Triathlon clothing is tight and slim cut because it actually *needs* to be. The bigger and baggier the clothing, the more "drag" in the water. Baggy clothing *will* get in the way.

For simplicity's sake, get thyself into a one-piece, sensible *swim*suit without skirts or shorts or tops. A one-piece ugly ole thing that holds you in and covers your boobage is just what the triathlon doctor ordered. (Yes, I am serious.)

Okay, so this one-piece "sensible" suit. The shoulder and back straps should be reasonably thick and supportive. If the suit "holds you in" and feels comfortable, then it's doing the job. If you are an average-size gal, something from a mainstream store will suit you just fine. The larger crowd (mine) may not fit into these brands. Although one-piece swimming suits are absolutely hideous and scream, "Watch out, here comes the newbie or tubby swimmer," I found a comfortable and practical tank suit at a plus-size clothing company.

> **Swim on the cheap:** an old one-piece tank swimsuit you've had forever; goggles ($15); swim cap ($5); borrowed/rented wetsuit for practices in open water, if necessary
>
> **Swim on the semicheap:** one-piece tank swimsuit ($65); goggles ($15); swim cap ($5); borrowed wetsuit for practices in open water
>
> **Swim like your bank account has no tomorrow:** one-piece tank swimsuit ($95); goggles, 2 pair ($60); swim caps ($20); wetsuit ($250); TriSlide lubricant ($12); kickboard ($30); fins ($50); paddles ($40); swim mesh bag ($20); hair care for swimming ($40)

Bike Gear

The bike: Many of us have a bike stashed in storage. Yes, the bike probably stinks and is old as all Christmas, but it might be enough to get you through for a bit. At the bare minimum, take the old bike to a bike store and get it adjusted to fit you as best as possible. If you have access to a cycling class at your gym, then you are in a good place to start training.

If your bike is a piece of crap, causes you physical pain to ride or feels "off," then you are probably in the market for a new(er) bike that fits you. Proper bike fit is monumental. The bike, of course, is your biggest investment, which is why I mentioned using the old dusty one in the garage for a bit. Still, a proper bike fit is something I cannot emphasize enough. From a motivational standpoint, if your bike is troublesome, you will hate the sport or think you are in worse shape than you might be. Therefore, investing in a reasonable bike should take high priority. Many bike stores carry used bikes, and the folks there can advise on your bike fit. Either way: get fitted.

If you're buying a bike, I recommend a *road* bike for a beginner. Tri bikes are expensive, and they can be hard to handle if you are new to cycling. If you can score a tri bike for a fraction of the original price, however, it might be worth the added difficulty. Otherwise, start with the cheaper, more beginner-friendly road bike—or even a hybrid.

Bike clothing: You need semifitted cycling clothing. A loose shirt will catch wind and have you sporting a parachute on your back. Fitted clothing is often horrifying. I still wear loose tops to indoor cycling class, but I proudly sport my stomach rolls in fitted jerseys and shorts when I am out on the roads cycling. I try to get away with a nice performance (wicking) shirt sometimes and some tighter shorts or capri pants on "fat" days. I am still very uncomfortable in very tight clothing, so I find what I can tolerate that still gives me the best performance.

For riding, padded shorts are a necessity. Pain on the Queen will deter your return to the bike. (Who is the Queen? If you can't figure it out, then ride an ill-fitting bike without padded shorts . . . and you'll learn.)

Regardless of what is covering my bum, you can bet that I am sporting some sort of padding in the shorts for the Queen. This padding is called a chamois ("shammy"). After a while in the bike seat (saddle), the Queen starts to hurt and grow grumpy from the pressure. Investing in a pair of chamois-padded shorts will make your cycling life more tolerable. The chamois pad will relieve some of this pressure and discomfort. Look for a one-piece pad, as it has fewer surface seams for chafing and pain.

If I had money to spend on a single piece of official triathlon clothing, for the initial investment, I would go with the chamois shorts. The padding makes the cycling experience much more enjoyable right out of the gate.

> **Bike on the cheap:** your old bike in the garage; a new helmet ($30–50); water bottle ($5); access to a gym with a cycling class ($75 a month); chamois-padded shorts ($50–75); an old tire pump
>
> **Bike on the semicheap:** an entry-level/used hybrid or road bike with bottle cage ($350); water bottles ($5); new helmet ($30–50); access to a gym with a cycling class ($75 a month); chamois-padded shorts ($50–75); bike pump ($25)
>
> **Bike like a fancy pants:** road bike or tri bike ($1,000–12,000) and saddle ($200); new helmet ($100–200); cycling shoes ($200–300); pedals ($100); water bottles ($15); rear bottle cage/hydration system ($40–150); bike bento box ($25); access to a gym with a cycling class ($75 a month); chamois-padded shorts ($90); pump ($50); tubes, CO_2 cartridges ($40); sunglasses ($100); bicycle trainer/indoor Spinning bike for house ($250–450); cycling jersey ($90); arm warmers ($30); power meter ($500); indoor virtual trainer ($1,000); "pain cave" indoor cycling equipment (computer, monitor, television, the works ($2,500); shoe covers ($30); cycling tights ($60); outer layer jacket ($100)

Run Gear

The shoes: Excellent running shoes are nonnegotiable. Find a running store in your town (or in the closest city). You should look for one of the places where the folks make you run on the treadmill while watching your gait, and where the employees look as if they stepped off a 20-mile trail run. These are the *loco* running people you can trust. Listen to what they say and buy what they recommend. Eight or nine times out of ten, they'll put you in a great shoe—and if not, they usually have great "run and return" policies if you have trouble with the fit.

I won't get into the great shoe debate: minimalist, stability, neutral, orthotics, inserts, barefoot, or the brands. Just go get a professional shoe fit and go from there. You will learn what makes your runs more comfortable, enjoyable, and injury-free. The best way to figure out which type of shoe you love is to run in different kinds of shoes. Just one word if you are heavier—don't let someone talk you into a minimalist or barefoot-style shoe. Starting out, the pounding will be too great on your body—you will want some sort of cushion on the bottom of your feet. Eventually, you may decide to transition to something more minimalist, but go slowly into this transition. And don't pick your shoes based solely on color.

Run socks: Good socks are like good shoes. If you purchase your shoes at a reputable running store, chances are that you will be offered some new socks. Get some good, synthetic-material socks (*not* cotton, whatever you do). And yes, at fifteen dollars a pair, most are worth it, as long as you have your sock-eating laundry monster under control. Give the monster a good talking to and get yourself some nice sockage.

Run clothing: Running is possible in virtually any clothing—just ask the firefighters who run full marathons in their fire garb. I prefer compression-style capri leggings for my bottoms, a good sports bra, and a semiloose-fitting wicking shirt. When I began running, though, I wore old T-shirts, shorts, and pants left over from weightlifting days. Like I said, you can get by with running in most anything.

I'm also a huge fan of sport-specific visors for running indoors and outside. The visor acts like a sweatband and is machine washable. Some women like hairbands. I didn't start out as a fan, but I am one now.

Additional gear: Another nice thing to have is a mini water bottle to carry on runs. I like the handheld ones for shorter runs and run-walks. The little snazzy bottle straps to your hand. As time passes and distances get longer for you, you may want to invest in a wearable belt or backpack hydration system, which can hold a ton of water and has pockets for keys, snacks, trinkets, and gels.

> **Run on the cheap:** sports bra ($20); excellent shoes and socks ($110)
>
> **Run on the semicheap:** sports bra ($40); excellent shoes and socks ($110); heart rate monitor ($90); running belt (to carry things) ($50)
>
> **Run through piles of cash:** sports bras ($100); *two* pairs of excellent shoes and many pairs of excellent socks ($220); GPS heart rate monitor ($200–500); wicking running shirts ($150); several pairs of running shorts ($150); running capris ($50); warm-up pants ($60); compression socks/sleeves ($60); visor ($25); running belt ($50); hydration system (bottles, belts, or backpack) ($75)

The Underpants Dance

We talked about training clothing and the importance of chamois, but we need to talk about our skivvies, too.

Bras: A well-fitting sports bra is necessary for keeping the Girls under control during all your biking and most importantly, running. You want some sort of wicking fabric to pull the moisture away from your skin. A pure cotton bra will retain moisture, which will *never* dry out in a race and can lead to chafing (you do not want chafing. Believe me. *The Girls do not want chafing*). Your bra should rein the Girls in, but also be comfortable.

When you are trying on bras, do the in-place jogging test. If you jog in-place and your boobs stay reasonably put, the bra feels good and you like it—then you have a good start. If you jump and your boobs knock the dressing room door open, find another one to try. The truth of the matter is that it's hard to tell if you have a good bra until you've worn it through a hard workout. When you find a good one, buy ten of them.

Underpants. Or not: If you are on the bike for long, underpants are a sworn enemy. A front wedgie on the bike is horrendous and will make you quit triathlon forever. Also, their seams will create even more issues for your parts. For now, if you want to wear underpants under your run shorts or pants or cycling shorts, go right ahead. But eventually, you'll be riding commando.

Yes, oh yes, yes, you will. Trust me.

Don't forget the lube: While we're talking underpants, don't forget lube. You do not want to chafe. Chafing is horrible, it's shocking how much it hurts, takes an ungodly amount of time to heal and thus, can be very discouraging. A standard lube, such as Aquaphor (or even whatever the up-to-date sports-specific lube is) helps significantly to prevent chafing. I use it under my arms or near my sports bra straps and bands. You can use this good stuff anywhere. On long bike rides and race days, I put it everywhere. I mean, *everywhere*, the Queen included. For getting started, it's nice to spread wherever something might be rubbing: skin on skin, sports bra on skin, and so on.

RACE DAY CLOTHING

The biggest triathlon mystery is *not* how to run. It is what to wear on race day. Race day clothing is a nightmare!

But here's the secret: find *one* thing to wear. Put it on before the swim. Then swim. Then bike. Then run. Then, take it off when you get home. Are you confused yet?* In a race, you should aim to wear a one-piece triathlon suit or a two-piece triathlon kit. A "kit" is usually a top and bottom combo that looks fancy. Regardless of whether you have a suit or a kit, your race day clothing is designed to be worn in all three stages of the race. In other words, you do not take it off!

Magic!

---

* Wearing one thing is the name of the game in shorter distance races, up to a half IRON-MAN. Once you are in Iron distance territory, all bets are off—just wear whatever in the world will get you to the finish.

With the exception of the wetsuit (if needed), you need not put *on* any other piece of clothing. This also means that you need not take *off* any clothing. You wear your wetsuit (again, only if needed) *on top* of your triathlon suit/kit. After the swim, you strip off the wetsuit, put on your helmet and cycling shoes, and are ready to go. You should never (ever) show your goodies in transition area.* Ever. Ever. The best way to avoid showing others your stuff is to keep your clothes *on*.

A triathlon suit/kit is typically made of a moisture-wicking material and has a pad in the shorts for cycling. The pad is thin, unlike the thick chamois pad for cycling, so you will want to spend some time on your bike wearing it ahead of time to get the Queen accustomed to less padding. But the thin pad allows the Queen's castle to dry much more quickly and not take on water like a diaper during the swim.

When you finish your swim, you will be soaking wet, this is true. But within a few minutes on the bike, you will find yourself almost dry. By the time you get to the run, you will not be thinking about your wet hair. This is the true beauty of the triathlon suit/kit. You may start out hating it, but eventually, you will love it. The darn thing is just so practical.

What if you cannot find anything to fit you (or that you would want to wear in public)? First of all, remember the *Slow Fat Triathlete* wisdom: *Do not care about what you look like when you are moving.* Worrying about how you look will undermine your ultimate goal—finishing the race. That being said, I understand. You may think, *I cannot wear this horrible-looking triathlon suit*. But you better do it, because if you are wearing something *different*, you will stand out much more than you would have imagined. And there are ways around it.

Triathlon Suit: One-Piece

A one-piece triathlon suit is typically a one-piece zip-up number that fits like a swimsuit with shorts attached. I like the one-piece suits because

---

*In longer-distance races (think: IRONMAN), there are changing tents—but that is because these races last from about 12 to 17 *hours*. You will not need to change clothes for a 1- to 4-hour event.

you need not worry about the top riding up and showing your belly. I also find that the one-piece compression suits hold in some of my jiggles.

The biggest negative with a one-piece suit is the difficulty to get in and out of it for bathroom purposes. But once you learn how to pee on the move (er, through your suit; yes, I'm sorry, it's true), you will not have to worry about that. My first suit ever is a one-piece and was purchased from an expensive company from a Google search.

You can spend $75–350 on a one-piece suit, depending on the brand and material (compression, pro-fabric, etc.).

Triathlon Suit: Two-Piece

Two piece "kits" are the most common deal on a race course. Traditional kits are slim cut and supertight—so they are tough for a larger-bodied woman or a beginner unaccustomed to spandex to even fathom wearing. But they sure are snazzy—yes, even on the Every Woman. And a kit has its many advantages: you can use the bathroom much easier; you can mix tops and bottoms; and you can look superfly.

The question of one-piece or two-piece is simply a matter of personal preference. You can spend $70–150 for *each* piece of a tri kit.

Do-It-Yourself Kit

Say you have a fitted wicking racer-back tank that you love and want to wear in the race. For example, a good choice is the Nike Women's Shape Sport Top, which goes up to plus sizes. If you have this top or something similar, you can always purchase a separate tri short to wear, and voilà! You will have a self-made kit of sorts.

Whichever top you choose, just remember, remember, remember— buy a *triathlon* short, *not* a *cycling* short to complete your kit. Any cycling short will turn into a swim diaper during the swim.

> **Race day on the cheap:** borrow a triathlon top and shorts, or get creative with your own do-it-yourself tri outfit (see "Race Day

Clothing Dos and Don'ts," which follows); borrowed/rented wet-suit, if necessary

Race day on the semi-cheap: discount tri shorts and top ($60); borrowed/rented wetsuit

Race day all-out: triathlon suit/shorts and top ($150–350); tran-sition mat ($30); gear bag ($75)

Race Day Clothing Dos and Don'ts

Do not wear new gear on race day. Do you really want to break in new shoes while running miles and miles? What if those supercute capris have a waistband that digs? You're stuck with them. So, again, *do not wear new gear on race day*. Not even socks. Give them a test run before race day.

Please, please do not wear a "real" bra anywhere near this race. Certainly do not wear your lacy underwire to the swim start as your do-it-yourself triathlon top. (I have seen this firsthand, or I would not write about it.)

Wear your sports bra under your tri suit during the swim if you have boobies bigger than a tabletop. Some suits or tops may have built-in sports bras, but seriously, unless you are teeny in the tatas, be careful. If your Girls are small and your suit has a built-in bra, then you *may* be good to go. Your headlights will likely be on during a race, so going without a bra can make the Girls shine like the top of the Chrysler Building. Keep in mind that while we (technically) do not care about what we look like while tri-ing, you *are* racing in essentially a wet T-shirt contest. I say, just put on your sports bra under your tri suit and forget about it.

Do not wear a one-piece *swim*suit to a tri unless you are: (1) a profes-sional triathlete; (2) plan to win the reace; or (3) you have tri shorts over it and intend to wear it for the entire race. A swimsuit plus tri shorts is a decent do-it-yourself tri kit. But if you can rock the swimsuit solo or wear a two-piece tri *bikini* for the entire race, then who's to stop you? Lawd, I applaud you, actually. The thought of *running* in a bikini makes my insides shiver.

I get questions all the time: *What if I wear my swimsuit during the swim, and then throw on my cycling shorts over it?* I am not going to say you can't do this, but keep in mind that you will be soaking wet after the swim and putting on tight shorts (while wet) is an Olympic event in itself. Weigh the pros and cons, and make your choice. But doesn't it sound easier to pick your one outfit—and just wear that?

My simple advice: do not change clothes during a race. Do not take anything (but your wetsuit) *off*. You can argue, and that's fine. But I still say no.

First, because changing clothes in transition is considered a newbie move and you will stand out like a sore thumb. While we don't (technically) care what people think about us (true), who really wants to stand out and look weird? Second, because it's truly impractical, frustrating (*Dry clothes! Wet body!*) and time consuming.

One caveat: In the beginning, I would throw on a T-shirt over my tri suit for the run only. I felt more comfortable that way and by the time I got to the run, I was dry. In hindsight, I looked silly. But at the time, it made me feel better. Sometimes you need to take care of your inner scaredy-cat in order to finish. If putting a T-shirt over your suit makes you feel better, then you should do it. If wearing a swimsuit and putting tri shorts over it makes you feel better, do it. You have to get to that starting line—that's the important thing! But please note that none of the above options involve *removing* clothing.

On race day, do not wear underpants. Really. They will not dry and you will end up with saddle sores on the Queen. Be nice to the Queen.

Do practice in your race day clothing well in advance of your race. Wear your race day suit to open water, cycling, and running. Make sure you like the fit, because the last thing you want is a clothing malfunction or discomfort on race day.

3 COACHING AND COMMUNITY

I T'S TRUE THAT TRIATHLETES *MAY* BE THE ONLY GROUP OF PEOPLE over the age of twenty-four who *do* have coaches, but you will be surprised (and in a good way) by the way a coach will change your motivation and your goals, and will set your mind at ease about training.

If you are not in a position to afford a coach, find a triathlon club or training group for accountability. First, you will enjoy your experience more if you are sharing it with others. Second, having others around will push you to do better and keep moving. Triathlon is a fabulous sport for community.

TAKING THE COACHING PLUNGE

On January 26, 2011, I became an official coached athlete. My coach was no stranger to me: Gerry. Cycling Instructor Extraordinaire.

My official training plan took off quickly. The first workout was a cycling class and a 2-mile run. (*What?!*)

I blinked and reread.

Workout 1: Spinning class

Workout 2: Two-mile run

So, I went to indoor cycling class and then I almost perished on a 2-mile treadmill run. *This coaching thing is not such a good idea after all,* I thought. Gerry just about killed me right out of the gate.

In triathlon, a "brick" workout is two of the disciplines back-to-back with a tiny break in between—just as you would have in a race. The idea behind a brick is to mimic actual race conditions. For example, a bike-run brick is hopping off your bike, lacing up your shoes, and going for a run. A swim-bike brick is jumping out of the pool, strapping on the helmet, and speeding off on the bike. The term *brick* is derived from the sensation in your legs when you begin running after cycling: your legs feel like complete bricks. (Personally, I think the term comes from the desire to throw a brick at your coach.)

But I did it. (The workout. I didn't throw a brick at Gerry.)

However, when I plugged my workout data into the training software, Gerry wrote me back: *NO no no. Not a brick, unless I tell you it's a brick.*

Oh, ooops. Yet another thing I learned. Two workouts, unless otherwise specified, just means two workouts sometime that day—not necessarily two back-to-back workouts. However, as I went along in the triathlon training process, I proceeded to brick absolutely everything. With job, kids, and schedule, I could not possibly have the luxury of two workouts a day. A morning and evening workout? *Puh-lease.* I had to do it all at once. I became a Brick House.

Coachly Things

Gerry was not an in-person coach. I saw him in cycling class, but mostly he formulated my training plan in three- to four-week blocks and sent me the workouts electronically. Usually, I read and questioned his sanity. Then, he told me to suck it up and to focus.

He has always been very nice to me. *Well, of course your coach should be nice to you,* you might say. But I know people who have crappy, mean-spirited coaches. People who pay their hard-earned money to be berated by superfast triathletes who have absolutely no humility (or humanity). I'm not sure I see the benefit derived from coachly abuse.

You can find almost any triathlete who might be willing to coach you—and for cheap. But do not fool yourself: you often get what you pay for, and the coach-athlete relationship *is* a relationship. You would not be friends with someone who was constantly mean. So, do not put up with a mean coach. Gerry was very *tough*, but he never was unkind to me.

You should benefit from and enjoy your coach-athlete relationship. Hopefully, your coach will feel the same way. At a minimum, a trust component must exist in your coaching relationship. You should feel comfortable enough to be honest with your coach about your physical abilities (and limits), your family situation(s), and your schedule. I trusted and still trust Gerry. He was with me from start to IRONMAN. Trust goes a long way.

Find Your Own Coach

Yes, having a coach costs money. Some coaches cost *a lot* of money. But sometimes, you'd be surprised—the cost per month for being a coached athlete is likely to be less than a few eating-out extravaganzas.

So . . . what should you look for in a coach?

Personality

For starters, find a coach who is a good match for you, personality-wise. Can you talk to her? Do you just plain like him? Believe me, "like" goes a long way. Facebook was on to something special with the Like button. Interview many coaches. Can you click Like . . . or do you want to scroll past or worse, unfriend?

Understanding Your Goals

If your coach believes you should be running a six-minute mile and you just started running yesterday, then she might not be the best coach for you. She might be a great coach, but simply not an ideal coach for a baby triathlete. Some coaches may have been tri-ing for so many years that they have lost a grip on what it means to run a thirteen-minute mile (on a good day).

Your coach should recognize your goals, no matter how crazy. But your coach should also understand your life, your family, and your (true) limitations. By "true" limitations, I mean your working hours, number of kids, and the like—not your lame-o excuses as to why you could "never" become a triathlete.

Empathy

I learned about Gerry's empathy up close and personal during my first open water swim and subsequent panic attack. Another coach would have likely given up on me on that day, in that cold water with my panic floating around in my wetsuit. Gerry was there to talk me through the fear; the empathy he showed me was incredible.

I recently thanked him for not giving up on me. He just shrugged his shoulders and said, "I have been there. I have had panic attacks in the water. I had to swim or be swum over. But I know how *absolutely* terrifying the open water swim *can* be. It's not a joke. It's real."

He continued, "But I also know that when an athlete faces her fears, there is an amazing energy there—it's like a drug—the energy itself is very uplifting. One of the reasons I like working with new triathletes is that they come to the sport absolutely scared to death. But during the process of training and racing, they find a way to dig down deep inside themselves. They are able to face their fears. Then, they find out: the scary dragon isn't that big."

A Catalyst

"I don't have any magic formula to my coaching," Gerry has explained to me. "I really simply try to bring *out* what is already *inside* the athlete. I'm not trying to put anything *into* the athlete—I'm trying to pull it *out*."

In other words, Gerry seeks to be a catalyst for his athletes.

"Triathlon is a servant, not a master—triathlon should be a means to self-discovery and self-actualization. It should *serve* your life, not *master* it."

Over the years I have seen athletes jump from coach to coach, blaming the coach for the reasons they are not succeeding at whatever goals they have. At the end of the day, it's up to the *athletes* to do the workouts, the work, and search and find for the greatness within themselves. The coach is truly a mentor, a catalyst; *that* is the role that works the magic.

Your End of the Bargain

Coached athletes have a duty to *try* not to drive their coaches up the wall. Note that I said "try." I mean, I *know* that I shouldn't call Gerry at three o'clock in the morning, freaking out about my run. So, I *try* not to call (sometimes I just e-mail and text six or sixteen times in a row).

We also have a duty of hard work. If you are paying money for a coach, then, for Pete's sake, pay attention to the coach and work hard. One of Gerry's biggest pet peeves? "I cannot stand an athlete's lack of ownership and 'buy-in' to the process. I do not like excuses. Saying the right words and not following through with the actions is a huge pet peeve, probably for any coach. I would prefer honesty. I would rather the athlete say, 'I *will not* do that workout,' rather than say, 'Yeah yeah, I will do that,' only to come up with an excuse later as to why it didn't get done. That is wasting *my* time and *their* money."

He said, "It's pretty simple. When I work with someone and they get beyond their limitations and it creates a snowball of energy and achievement—that's why I coach."

Join a Triathlon Club or Team

As a beginner, a local triathlon club or team may be just what you need to get moving. For starters, you will immediately meet some of the craziest people in your area (the triathletes). Once you join a club, you may have access to coaching, training programs, group rides, and events (oh, and fancy triathlon suits for races!). Joining a triathlon club will give you the accountability factor that otherwise might be missing.

Additionally, if you can't stand the thought of training alone, this is *definitely* the way to go. Joining a triathlon club can be a really intimidating place as a beginner. Remember that a club or team is like a pair of running shoes—they might be beautiful and wonderful, but they may also not fit you. You need to find what works for you—and don't give up if someplace doesn't feel right. Somewhere *will*. Keep looking.

Organizations, such as Team in Training (www.teamintraining.org) provide coaching and training in exchange for fund-raising. If you are interested in making a difference *while* you learn to tri, you might benefit from Team in Training or a similar organization.

4 SAFETY AND SMARTNESS

BEFORE WE DIVE INTO THE NITTY-GRITTY OF TRIATHLON, I BEG a commitment from you. I want you to promise that as you embark on triathlon and training that you will:

Be Smart
Be Safe
Become a Student

BE SMART

One definition of *smart* is to be "mentally alert." At all times during your training, you should practice mental alertness. You must be cognizant of your surroundings, your body, and your mind.

Part of the challenge, especially as a beginner, is to keep tabs on your technique, your energy levels, and your health. Make sure that you are feeling okay during your training sessions. At the same time, you must be smart and remember that hard work is the only path to success in your triathlon goals. *Does it really hurt, or are you just uncomfortable with the heat and the sweat? Can you push through and finish that last half mile?* Be smart and know your limits, but at the same time, give yourself some credit and do not let your mind tell your body, "I can't," when it certainly can.

Working hard and suffering through sweat is one thing, but heart palpitations and serious pains are another. If your knees feel as if someone has busted them with sledgehammers, then stop running. If you are bleeding from the head, then you should stop pedaling (or at least slow down). If you are dizzy, sick, vomiting, pooping on yourself . . . call it a day. If you don't sleep well before a long ride and you feel nauseated in the morning, you must gauge whether you are capable of pushing through, or whether you think pushing would be dangerous to your health.

More often than not, you can push through it—*and* you will be just fine. But every so often, you will be exhausted and ill and need a break. Learn to listen to your body, but don't let your body give you lame excuses either.

Be smart in your training and the smarts will translate to a safe and healthy race day. Even if not, it will make the odds be ever in your favor. (Really? Did you think I would omit a perfectly timed reference to *The Hunger Games?*) Gerry says that some of the stupidest triathlon decisions are made because someone is overtired on race day. Your mental alertness is important for your own safety and the safety of others.

BE SAFE

In recent times, female runners have been experiencing a targeting of sorts by sickos who want to assault our athletic kind. Do not run in the dark on a deserted road. Do not run in the wee hours of the morning without a headlamp. Preferably, do not run alone. If you are out alone, do not wear ear buds. Carry pepper spray. Learn self-defense. Being safe goes back to being smart. If you feel scared on a run, go home. Nothing is worth your life. Until the world changes, here we are.

Wear a safety ID bracelet or have your ID close on your person. A wearable safety ID is easy, because it's *on* you: a bracelet, anklet, or shoe fob that contains your personal information, such as name, date of birth, and drug allergies, in addition to emergency contact information. I consider this a necessity.

Of course, we cannot control the actions of others. But aim to place yourself in the safest environments possible. Ride on low-traffic streets. Run in well-traveled and well-lit areas. Never swim in the open water alone. While these safety measures won't absolutely protect you from the idiots in this world, they may lessen the chance that the idiots will find you.

Yes, this a fun book, but triathlon safety is no joke. A swim course can be tough and dangerous. Running in the dark, when you can't see and others can't see you, is dangerous. A bike is dangerous. You must learn how to ride your bike. You must learn the rules of the road *and* the race. You must wear your helmet. You must not ride in "packs" on a triathlon race course. You must *not* wear your ear buds while riding a bike. *Ever. Do you hear me? What? You can't hear me because you're wearing your ear buds? Oh, I see . . .*

BECOME A STUDENT OF TRIATHLON

You may think, *I can't do a race because I can't ride a bike.* Unfortunately, that has not stopped some people. And I do not mean that in a good way.

It is fine if you cannot ride a bike *today*. You will learn. But you should *not* go to your first triathlon if you cannot ride your bike comfortably and safely. If you cannot pedal in a straight line, wait until you *can* before you participate in a race. If you cannot shift gears, wait. I will cheerlead, "You can do a triathlon," until you are sick of hearing me, but you will *never* hear me tell you to just go out and try one without some experience, smarts, and safety.

I am a firm believer in becoming a student of triathlon. Even though I ran out and did my first tri pretty quickly, I had absorbed and read a ton of books, blogs, and magazines beforehand. I had ridden that evil bike in the past. I knew how to pump my tires, change a tube, and fix a dropped chain. I was bad with clipping in and out of my pedals, but only to my own detriment (stopping and going). Once I was in the pedals, I knew and followed the rules. I knew that you must stay to the right of the road, not draft and pass within so many seconds, and announce, "On Your Left!" when passing.

I hope that the upcoming sections on the swim, bike, and run will guide you through your training, race preparation, and race day. Remember to read the USA Triathlon rules for sanctioned events and spend some time devouring articles on swim starts, bike handling, and race courtesies.

It's simple: just read, learn, and absorb the safety measures and rules. Even when you may not be fast or close to it, you will at least be a good student of triathlon and you'll be on your way. Your family will thank you—because you'll be around to see more days of racing. And your fellow racers will thank you. More than you know.

5 A BRIEF INTERLUDE ON DATA

I DO NOT WANT TO OVERWHELM YOU WITH DATA AND NUMBERS. You may already be familiar with data—which is great. But you may not. So, I would be remiss in my job here if I glazed over the importance of some data for training, especially if you want to keep going in the sport.

If numbers make you cringe and think, "I just can't with all this data and details!"—then go ahead and skip to Chapter 6. Seriously. Just know that at some point, the data *will* become relevant if you continue to advance or if you want to get faster, better, and stronger.

Now, for the data junkies—here is your first dip in the water.

HEART RATE

Heart rate training for building your endurance is a cornerstone of the bike and the run. Why? What is your heart rate good for?

When I began to bike and run, my heart felt as if it would explode. This is one of the most common mistakes with beginners—we think that all "working out" is redlining. While we certainly *can* work out really hard, that is actually not the greatest way to start out. This is where the heart rate becomes important. (Well, the heart rate is always important—but here is where we pay mind to it.) Cycling and running too fast and too hard (and too frequently) puts athletes (new and experienced) at risk for injuries, exhaustion, and burnout.

We have certain "zones" for your heart rate—typically from Zone 1 (easy) to Zone 5 (hardest), and these are set personally for you through testing of your lactate threshold. For the purpose of simplicity, this is the transition phase between aerobic (with oxygen) and anaerobic (without oxygen) work in training. When you use heart rate training to build endurance, you are essentially teaching your muscles to use oxygen more efficiently, and thus the less lactic acid will be produced. Translation: endurance increases, running and biking feel easier, and therefore you will go faster and be fitter.

You can measure your heart rate in many ways—technology is always advancing in this field—from chest straps to wrist straps to built-in monitors in watches and data that upload to our phones and training programs.

One of the most important things to remember, however, is that most devices have preset "zones" in the watch or monitor; it is up to you to input *your* proper training zones. Do not rely on the factory settings.

Okay. We will talk more about heart rate training within bike and run.

CADENCE AND STROKE RATE

Cadence is simply a term used to describe the turnover of your feet—on the pedals on your bike, or the foot strikes on the ground in your run. In your swim, you might hear *cadence* used, but usually the term is *turnover* or *stroke rate*.

Generally speaking, the faster your cadence or stroke rate, the faster you will travel across sea and land. The key is finding the balance between speed in your turnover and effort in your output. In other words, you need an easy enough resistance/effort to be *able* to have a faster cadence. Cadence improves with time and practice.

For the easiest and most delicious analogy, think about stirring a spoon through water versus through peanut butter. You can easily swish it in the water and go faster and faster, improving your cadence with relative ease. Eventually your arm or wrist might tire out, but it will take a while. In the peanut butter, however? Well, nothing to do there but eat that. Turning a spoon in peanut butter, especially chunky and organic, will really tire a gal out. So, as you see, the lower the resistance, the better the cadence.

Cadence will be discussed in more detail in the bike and run sections.

PACE AND SPEED

Some may disagree with me wholeheartedly on this, but I believe as a true beginner to swim, bike, or run—or all—it's best to throw the measurement of pace (e.g., your speed) completely out the window for whatever sport you are new to.

I believe this for a few reasons. First, pace is something that this entire sport is measured by. There is plenty of time to worry about it. If you are new to a discipline, then just don't fret about the speed you are going. For now, we are just moving and working toward a goal. I would, at the very least, challenge you to not worry about pace for the first two months in your training.

Next, pace will improve with time and consistency. Once you have spent some time moving forward and being consistent, then you can begin to measure pace.

Finally, pace will make you feel like crap if you are a slow beginner. You will begin to look at everyone else, begin the nasty comparison game, and—unless you are really strong of mind and spirit—this can be a big downer and potentially an excuse to quit. If you think pace and speed are a detriment, just don't worry about them.

Seriously. Forward *is* a pace. Sometimes, it's the only pace that matters. I have taken some heat over the years for how "slow" I am. But time and time again as I finish 70.3 and IRONMAN races within the time cutoffs and without quitting, I continue to tout that forward is a pace. If you work hard and do what is best for you, then forward is the only pace that matters. Be proud.

When you are ready, then start to work on your speed. You will know when that time is right. Give yourself the space to grow into it.

POWER

For our purposes, power is a cycling measurement. Power on the bike is a measurement of output by the rider. Your bike power is measured by a power meter—a device attached to your bike that measures the output of *you* on the bike. The meter works by using a gauge that deflects when a force is applied—so it measures torque and combines with angular velocity—and gives the power "watts" of the output. Cycling with power can be considered an advanced methodology for triathlon that is covered in only slightly more detail in the bike section of this book. Cycling with a power meter will *not* make you faster—but it will give you the state of things. What you choose to do with that data? (Ride more, train harder, nothing?) Well, that's what makes you faster (or not).

6 THE SWIM

I ENJOY SWIMMING FOR THE MOST PART. IF YOU DO NOT ENJOY swimming, then go ahead and start repeating to yourself: *I love to swim. I love to swim. I love to swim.* The vast majority of triathlon success (and failure) may be attributed to your mental strength. So start tricking your mind into loving it now!

Really, swimming really *is* a wonderful thing.

A common saying for triathlon swimming is: *You cannot win a triathlon in the swim, but you can certainly lose it.* Practicing the swim is vitally important for many reasons. First, it is quite dangerous to slack on the swim. In cycling and running, you can stop moving, get off your bike, or stop running and slow to a walk. In swimming, you better keep swimming or . . . well, you know.

Second, the swim start in a race is often crowded and full of intense energy. The goal of the triathlon swim should be to feel comfortable in the water and also, to swim strongly to avoid fatigue going into the next part of the race. The more relaxed and less fatigued you are coming out of the water, the better your overall race will be. If you begin a race completely terrified, with your heart racing and your mind blown, you are creating a dangerous environment for yourself and others (not to mention a likely bad race).

Finally, I beg you to learn to love the water. How? By convincing yourself that you do! When I was a teenager in Olympic weightlifting, my training included one lift that I hated to do. Hated it. I would dread those particular days. Each day on the drive to the gym, my mom would say, "Tell yourself that you love it!"

I would roll my fifteen-year-old eyes at her, thinking, *What does she know?*

But I began to repeat "I love this lift, I love this lift" to myself before each training session. Eventually, that particular lift became my *best* and *favorite* lift. Gerry's triathlon advice is to use your *mind* to control your *body*. Turns out, my dear momma started me on this brilliant training even before the triathlon came into the picture.

I WAS GOING TO SWIM!

I will never forget the first day of swimming as a baby triathlete in training. I had been a part of a swim team in my younger years, so I strapped on my swim cap and thought, *Oh yeah, here I come again! Watch out! Taking on the swim world!* But I had no recollection of how to really swim. After slapping myself in the face about sixteen times while trying to put on my nonsilicone, hair-tearing swim cap and situating the cap over my ears, under my ears, then over again (*is this right?*), I was ready. I was wearing my new plus-size swimsuit. I wore my fancy new goggles (*over my cap, right?*).

I eased myself down into the pool, scraping my back in the process. I went under, pushed myself off the wall with my feet, and began to flail through the water. After five strokes, I stood straight up in the lap lane— not even halfway down the pool. I could not breathe and my heart was absolutely racing. *What in the . . . ?* I went back underwater and tried to swim to the end of the pool. I finally made it, and I grabbed onto the pool wall, struggling for air.

To say I was shocked would be an understatement. *Had I ever swum at all? Swim team? Hello?? What in the . . .*

That day in the pool was an opportune time to give up. To think I would ever swim in a triathlon seemed impossible. But I spent that morning swimming wall to wall, resting, struggling for breath, catching my breath, and then starting again.

The next swim workout, I was able to do a little more. And with each workout . . . a tad more, and more.

Swimming may feel like the most evil discipline of triathlon when you start. But something is very interesting about swimming. Even if you can't swim a lick right now, you will see *big* fitness gains almost immediately In the pool— more so than on the bike or the run. Trust me: in a few short weeks, you will see your swim workout go from a pitiful 100 yards to a decent (but slow) 500 yards. A month or so after that, you'll be swimming 1,500 yards without dying, and you will be amazed.

The swim stroke you want to learn is the traditional *freestyle* stroke, also known as the front crawl. The front crawl is (should be) the fastest of all stroke options (as opposed to breaststroke or backstroke), although you *are* permitted to swim however you'd like in a race. You will, however, be disliked by others as a breaststroker. The front crawl basically consists of using your arms, in alternating front forward motions, to *pull* and *crawl* yourself through the water. Sometimes you may feel so terrible swimming, the *crawl* terminology is eerily symbolic. The arm stroke is made up of three primary movements known as the recovery, catch, and pull. As your arms rotate, each arm goes through the motion of *recovery, catch*, and *pull*.

I will not waste time *describing* the mechanics of the swim. The very best way to learn how to swim will not come from *reading*. I recommend lessons (if you have no idea how to swim), then master's class (described later in this section), and watching videos of proper swim technique. Then (brace yourself), watch videos of yourself swimming *and* have an experienced swimmer watch you or your clips.

———— SWIM DISTANCE CHEAT SHEET ————

One length of a standard gym pool is either 25 yards or 25 meters. A yard pool is shorter than a meter pool. Ask your gym manager which length pool is available.

A "length" means swimming from one end to another.
Wall |— ⇨—| Wall
= One Length

Swimming from one end to the other and returning to the start is one "lap."
Wall |— ⇨—| Wall
Plus
Wall |— ⇨—| Wall
= One Lap

25-meter pool
Quarter mile: 16.1 lengths; 8 laps
Half mile: 32.2 lengths; 16.1 laps
One mile: 64.4 lengths; 32.2 laps

25-yard pool
Quarter mile: 17.6 lengths; 8.8 laps
Half mile: 35.2 lengths; 17.6 laps
One mile: 70.4 lengths; 35.2 laps

THE SWIM FOR THE EVERY WOMAN

Megan Melgaard
Fix My Swim
www.FixMySwim.com

Megan Melgaard has led an eclectic aquatic life—from winning US National and Masters World Championships, conducting water safety exercises for Delta Airlines, and racing around islands. After years of pursuing her dreams in swimming, she was awarded a college scholarship and a spot on the US National Team. Megan has raced a plethora of on- and off-road triathlons, including an IRONMAN and age-group podium at XTERRA Off-Road World Championships. She has even been seen in a Hollywood stunt car and acting alongside Ashton Kutcher and Kevin Costner in 2006's The Guardian, where she played a Coast Guard rescue swimmer in training—not many people can say that, eh? The self-professed "Aquapreneur" with over twenty years' experience is a swim instructor and consultant through her company Fix My Swim, while serving full-time as director of events for Swim Across America, a nonprofit.

The swim might be one of the biggest barriers to doing a triathlon. Preparation for the swim portion of your triathlon is of paramount importance because the open water environment is dynamic, differing greatly based on location, experience, and conditions. The primary goal is to have a safe and successful swim—so, let's go!

First, assess your swimming background and experience level. Were you a strong swimmer growing up and on a swim team? Have you been out of the water for a while and just need to dust off your goggles? Is your most recent swimming accomplishment doing the doggy paddle across the resort pool? Regardless of background, the wonderful thing about swimming is that it welcomes all levels and ages.

Once you assess your level, consider where you fit into one of three categories: beginner/newbie, intermediate, or advanced. Work on proper technique and build stamina with a combination of drill, endurance, and/or interval workouts to help you prepare for your specific race distance.

Aim to swim three or four times a week as your schedule allows, as frequency is your friend for best results. A program, group training, or preplanned set of workouts can help you achieve your goal of a successful swim. Train and familiarize yourself in the open water environment. Make sure you are able to swim the distance of your target race (without breaks!) well before race day.

Beginners and Newbies

Learning how to swim with proper technique should be your main priority. Research a local adult Learn-to-Swim program, triathlon training group, or private coach in your area. Find a coach or program that currently works with beginner adult swimmers. Explain that you are new to swimming with a goal of completing your first triathlon and discuss whether a group or one-on-one session might work best for you.

Freestyle

As you embark upon your swimming journey, your primary focus should be on freestyle. Freestyle, also known as the front crawl, is the fastest, most efficient, and preferred stroke amongst triathletes. While the other nonfreestyle strokes (breaststroke, backstroke, and butterfly) may be performed, remember that freestyle is your mainstay for race day.

When learning freestyle, there are a few main elements to focus upon:

Body Position

Maintain a horizontal body position with activated core (midsection) for greatest efficiency.

Practice the following exercise: in the pool, push off the wall in an area where you will be able to stand. Outstretch both arms in the front, spine in a neutral position, and bring the legs together. Glide after pushing off the wall, while keeping a taut core to maintain a horizontal body position. When your speed slows, stand up.

Breathing

When starting out, breathe to your dominant side—whichever side feels most comfortable.

Eventually you should learn to breathe bilaterally (on both sides). Bilateral breathing involves breathing every third stroke, helping with balance and situational awareness. Unilateral breathing is also widely accepted, as long as you maintain symmetrical body rotation and proper form. Unilateral breathing may benefit you in certain situations, such as waves coming from one direction, where it behooves you to breathe to the opposite side.

Consider training *bilaterally* and racing *unilaterally*. Discuss with your coach or team, if applicable, what may be the best breathing method for you.

Practice the following exercise: while standing on the bottom of the pool, bend at the waist and outstretch your nondominant arm. With the nondominant arm, hold onto the end of a kickboard or the wall and place your head in the water looking down. Turn your head and breathe to the opposite, or dominant side, then return your head to the water. Practice breathing in and out, with a relaxed inhale and exhale. If you feel you are not getting enough air, relax and take in a deeper breath, but be careful of "vacuuming" in too much air or spending excess time in the breathing position. If you are feeling discomfort with the exhale, pretend you are breathing out of a straw or simply sigh the air out.

It is important to keep the nondominant arm outstretched when breathing for stability and lift. Pressing the arm down while breathing will cause you to lose lift, increase drag, and present a more difficult breathing position.

Arm Movements

The arm should enter the water at a slight angle and extend forward before pulling. Move through the phases of the underwater stroke: the "catch," acceleration, and finish.

The catch will initiate water moving backward in the beginning of the stroke. Your elbow will be a lever while your palm faces backward, not down. Elbow position stays "up," or higher than your wrist.

The acceleration phase utilizes arm, back, and core muscle groups, synchronized with body rotation to produce a powerful motion underneath your body. With your palm still facing backward, the pull movement will create a small S-shape trajectory, coming under your hip area and exiting near or just past your thigh area. From the point your hand/arm enters the water to the exit, be careful not to cross over your body's center line.

The finish will further push your body forward. Upon recovery, your hand should stay relaxed while moving quickly forward over the water in preparation to reenter the water and initiate the next stroke.

Kick

A proper kick will aid in propulsion, balance, and rotation. The slight kick movement should come from your hip area and not from your knee or calf. Relax your ankles and gently point your toes to effectively kick the water backward. For triathlon, maintain a soft, rhythmic kick and take care not to kick too much, which will expend valuable energy. Note that when wearing a wetsuit, you will likely kick less due to the neoprene's limiting your movement.

Kick Drill Exercise: Superman Kick

How: Your arms stay in the front balanced extended position, shoulder width apart. Maintain flexible leg kicking, using hip flexors and quads, and allow your hips to slightly rock back and forth while kicking. Stop, raise your head, or take a regular arm stroke to breathe. You can also do this exercise with a board, extended out front and breathe to the side with a stroke, or forward per your preference.

Safety Stroke

Make sure to learn a safety or "rest" stroke to rely upon when swimming in open water. (More information on safety strokes is provided later in this chapter.)

A personalized approach and instruction from a qualified coach will help you understand swimming fundamentals so you can progress more quickly and avoid potential injury. Also, a variety of swimming videos are available online.

Intermediate Swimmers

If you have a background in swimming, yet haven't been in the water recently, consider joining a local swim program, triathlon club, or US Masters Swimming Program. This will be the single greatest thing you can do for your swim as an intermediate swimmer.

Swimming with a group or club provides the opportunity to help you gauge your endurance level, hone skills, and build speed through structured workouts. While it might seem intimidating, there are programs for all swimming levels. A group or club is a great way to connect and train with others who share similar goals. Here are some tips when jumping into your first group practice:

Establishing a Lane

Upon arrival, introduce yourself and share your goals, as well as swimming level, with the coach. The coach will place you in the appropriate lane for the workout for your skill level.

Workouts

Sessions begin with a warm-up, followed by "sets," which are a series of swim distances separated by time intervals, or rest periods. Coaches may incorporate drills and provide technique suggestions during the workout. Ask the coach for one specific element or drill that you can focus on each week. Make sure to warm down to be better prepared for your next workout.

Circle Swimming

When there are multiple people in a lane, swimmers travel down the right side of each length, thus swimming in a counterclockwise direction. This is referred to as circle swimming.

Passing

The technique to pass in a lane is to give a light tap on the foot of the swimmer you are passing. If tapped, pull over closer to the lane line while swimming or stop at the end of the length to let the other swimmer pass.

Advanced Swimmers

If you have been swimming for quite some time and are familiar with racing in the pool and/or open water, you are ready to start at the front of the pack! As an advanced swimmer, you may want to focus more on speed and racing techniques.

Practice Race-Specific Workouts

Mimic the heart rate pattern often seen in a race by doing such sets as the following, where the number of 100s depends on the specific race distance:

> 20 x 100s with: 10–15 seconds rest
>
> 1–2 90% effort
>
> 3–19 steady race pace: 10–15 seconds rest
>
> 20 build the kick and exit the pool (be sure to raise your body to vertical gradually, to avoid a heart rate spike or lightheaded feeling)
>
> Warm down

Practice Drafting

Many fast swimmers will be able to find "clean" water out in front; though most may find themselves in a "pack" of swimmers or in close proximity to others. "Drafting" is a useful tool to save energy in the swim when the opportunity presents itself.

Immediately behind: This method is often referred to as "pace line" drafting. Stay within 1 to 2 feet of the swimmer in front of you to reap the benefit of less drag and greater efficiency. Take care not to hit the person's feet in front of you (to avoid being kicked) and ensure that the swimmer in front of you knows where they are going! This method may require you to sight higher; over the person in front of you to see the buoy.

Slightly to the side: Drafting behind a swimmer and slightly to the side or closer to the lower half of the leg will allow you to breathe and sight more effectively. This method offers less drag than drafting in a pace line.

On the hip: If you find yourself close to another competitor and can draft off the person's hip (your shoulder will be in line with the swimmer's hip), you will gain an even greater advantage than drafting on the feet or by the lower leg.

Every Woman Swim Drills

Even if you are a beginner, you can benefit from the practice of "drills." Drills help you focus on and strengthen certain aspects or elements of the swim stroke. Some example drills include: Catch Up Series, Doggy Paddle, and Push the Pool.

Catch Up Series: Superman, Accelerated, and Kickboard
Superman Catch Up

Focus: Horizontal body position, stability, and lift while breathing.

How: Start with your hands/arms in the front extended position, shoulder width apart. Stroke with one arm, while your opposite arm stays extended in the front. Concentrate on leaving your nondominant breathing arm out, then engaging in a strong pull once your head is back in the water after the breath. Utilize a strong core connection. Match your arms back in the front of the stroke and begin the pull with your opposite arm. Timing is important. This drill should be done slowly with focus on balance, while rotating your body through each stroke.

Accelerated Catch Up

Focus: Find synchronicity in this drill between the extended "gliding" arm, catch, and rotation of your body as your arm passes through the acceleration phase of the stroke. When breathing, maintain nondominant arm position by not letting it "push" or drop down too quickly.

How: Stroke with one arm, while your opposite arm stays in the front extended position. Timing is different from Superman Catch Up in that you should move your extended arm *just before* the opposite arm has met the other arm in the front extended position. Focus on rotation with a strong core connection and full follow-through of the stroke.

Catch Up with a Kickboard
For Beginners

Use this drill if you need to slow things down or are having trouble with timing with Catch Up or matching your arms in the front.

Focus: Train the arm on your nonbreathing side to remain in the horizontal position, rather than pushing down on the water to "help" you breathe. Your arm should stay out in a balanced extended position. Concentrate on a strong pull and good core connection.

Equipment: Kickboard

How: This is very close to the one-arm drill with the board, from above, yet you are using both arms. Start with both hands on the bottom of the board. Swim with one arm at a time, while your other arm is holding onto the bottom of the board. Slow down the stroke and focus on one arm at a time, repeating with both arms.

Doggy Paddle

Focus: Fun and functional, Doggy Paddle will help develop the catch phase of the stroke, build strength, and give awareness of moving and controlling the water early on in the stroke.

How: Your head can be above or below water, while your arms stay underwater at all times. While keeping your head steady, look forward, or down if you would like to watch your hand movements. Use a slight kick to maintain a horizontal body position. Fully extend one arm to the front (in front of your shoulder) with a slight body rotation. Akin to curling over the water or rolling your arm over an exercise ball, bend your elbow into a vertical forearm position, as the palm of your hand moves the water backward. Finish near the midtorso while your other arm repeats the same movement. Slide your arm back up to the full extension position and pull again.

Push the Pool

Focus: This drill focuses on the finish, or push phase, of the stroke. Keeping your body firm and straight, feel the propulsion generated from the push and force on the water through the finish phase.

How: Perform regular freestyle. While moving through the acceleration phase in normal fashion, push through the end of the stroke as your palm faces the back wall. Hold in this position for a beat (short second) to "ride" the push and effort of the finish/follow-through. (Think of giving someone a high five in the back of the stroke.) Feel some of the water pass by your thigh, rather than into your thigh, for correct placement.

Open Water Dynamics

Most triathlon swims take place in what is called open water: a wide variety of options, including lakes, oceans, seas, rivers, canals, bays, and more. Open water swimming is wonderfully dynamic, and no two swims will ever prove to be alike. Adapting yourself to the environment will be your key to success, as each body of water will present different conditions.

Open water swimming differs from a controlled pool setting in clarity, temperature, depth, and surface activity, to name a few. It is very important to experience open water swimming *before* your first target race. Start by swimming with an experienced swimmer or group that is familiar with local waters. Investigate water and weather conditions prior to jumping in. Ultimately, the more you know, the more prepared you will be. As you progress and gain confidence, practice in different conditions, such as wind and waves, to be ready for whatever comes your way on race day.

When Starting Out in Open Water

Start slow. One of the first things you will want to do is literally get your feet wet. Walk the shoreline to learn what the bottom comprises (rock, sand, mud, etc.), as well as the slope or incline. By doing this, you can assess where it is safe to jump or walk in to begin your swim.

There are no lane lines or walls to rest upon, so make sure to start slowly and swim in an area where you can stand, offering a safe opportunity to take a break if needed. Begin with short swims and gradually increase your distance as you become more comfortable. Find and maintain a stroke rhythm that works for you.

Know YOUR Safety Stroke

A safety stroke is one that you can revert to at any point during training or racing in open water so as to comfortably regain composure midswim, should you become tired, anxious, or disoriented. Sometimes, performing a few strokes or taking a moment to regroup will help calm the nerves. Practice your preferred safety stroke in the pool.

Safety strokes include treading water, the head-up breaststroke, side-stroke, traditional backstroke, or float.

With the float stroke, you can roll onto your back for a few seconds and kick. Resting or floating on your back is a convenient way to catch your breath without movement. Try counting backward from 10 to 1 while calming the breath. When ready to return to freestyle, raise your arm above your head (as if you are answering a question in grade school), turn onto your stomach, and perform the initial pull with that same arm to reestablish your stroke. Kicking on your back also provides an opportunity to reach up and clear out foggy goggles.

───────── NEVER SWIM ALONE. ─────────

Always swim with a friend, coach, or group. In addition to safety and account-ability, they can help provide confidence in the water, tips, and fun.

Sighting in Open Water

Sighting, sometimes referred to as spotting, is a critical technique in open water swimming. Without the assistance of lane lines and markings seen on the bottom of the pool, sighting will help you stay on course.

When sighting in a triathlon, you will target and swim toward a "mark" or "buoy." Buoys used in races are usually round or tetrahedron-shape inflatables and are brightly colored. Turn buoys (where you make a turn or change course) are often a different color than directional course buoys. Study the course and directions given in the pre-race briefing. The easiest way to swim is to sight and swim from buoy to buoy until complete.

Tips for Sighting

Keep moving. Sighting is best when combined with a stroke, as it is important to maintain a horizontal body position and continue advancing forward.

Use alligator eyes. While your arm is extended out to the front in the beginning of the stroke, keep holding that same arm straight out and quickly raise your eyes ("pop your goggles") above the surface of the water. This is the "alligator eyes" method of sighting.

Try to sight every six to ten strokes—maybe more on a technical course, maybe less on a straight swim with lots of people—just depends.

Time your breath. There are several methods to integrate the breathing movement with sighting: (1) breathe as normal to the side, then turn your head to the front for the sight; (2) pop the goggles above the surface for "alligator eyes," then turn your head for the breath; or (3) sight independently from your breath, which is taken during the next stroke sequence. You'll want to avoid breathing to the front, as this will result in poor body position and increased drag. Breathing to the front can also cause you to get water in your mouth, especially in rougher water conditions.

Study the landscape. Evaluate the course and buoy placements before the swim begins. If conditions, such as sun glare or fog, present visual challenges, identify landmarks or features beyond the buoys to sight on, as they will help guide you in the right direction. Before embarking on your swim, assess how the water is moving. Lake water is usually flat, resulting in a calm surface, making it easy to sight. Ocean conditions may require you to sight higher than usual to see over waves or chop. Rivers may also have currents, requiring you to adjust your trajectory from point A to point B.

Equipment
Wetsuit

First things first: water temperatures vary based on location, weather, and the body of water itself. On race day, site-specific temperatures will dictate whether you can wear a wetsuit. A wetsuit is never required. USA Triathlon (USAT) rules will provide the cutoff temperature for the wetsuit and whether it isn't allowed for awards, so remember to check your race and USAT rules.

A wetsuit provides warmth and insulation, as well as buoyancy and compression. What this means for you is the potential for better body position, increased speed, and greater efficiency in the water.

A triathlon wetsuit is specific to the sport (different from, say, a diving wetsuit). It has a slick exterior to reduce water resistance and drag, resulting in superior hydrodynamics compared to a suit made for scuba diving or surfing.

Proper fit is essential! You need to make sure that the suit is comfortable for you, especially in the neck and chest area. A suit that is too tight may cause decreased mobility or restricted breathing. A loose wetsuit may fill with water and cause unnecessary drag. Whether to have a suit with full sleeves or one that is sleeveless is a personal preference, though full sleeves are most common.

When choosing your suit, consider the temperature of the water where you will be training and racing. A full-sleeve wetsuit will offer more warmth by providing additional coverage. When evaluating options, consider a suit that offers thinner neoprene around the shoulder area. Sleeveless wetsuits, by nature, will allow for more shoulder and arm flexibility. Ensure a good fit between the body and armpit area to avoid gaps, which may allow unwanted water to enter the suit. Be sure to practice with your wetsuit in open water before race day. You may also want to rehearse unzipping and getting out of the wetsuit for faster T1 (transition) times.

Safety tip: Wetsuits are not considered lifesaving devices. Use caution in cold water for conditions related to hypothermia. In warm water, be aware of conditions related to hyperthermia or heat illness.

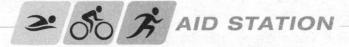

TECHNIQUES FOR PUTTING ON THE WETSUIT

Purchase Body Glide, TriSlide (spray), or a similar balm to help the wetsuit go on easier. BodyGlide will also help prevent chafing. Common areas to apply are around your neck and under your arms.

continues

> *continued*
>
> Place plastic bags on your feet. While sitting, hold the suit in front of you with the zipper in the back. Slide your legs through the suit, then remove the bags from your feet. While standing, slowly pull the suit up to your knees, then roll or gently pull up the suit from the inside, above your thighs and waist, then up to your torso and arms. (Akin to pantyhose!) Use the pads of your fingers to pull up the suit to prevent nicks or punctures of the neoprene. Be aware of jewelry or sharp objects that may also tear the suit. Zip up the suit via the string attached to the zipper or have someone help you.

Swim Cap

Swim caps are made of latex, silicone, or fabric. Many swimmers choose to train in silicone caps, a slightly thicker and softer material than latex, which won't pinch or pull your hair. Latex caps are typically provided to participants at races. For greater visibility in open water, it's best to choose a bright color (think hot pink, neon green, or yellow) for visibility from boats or by other swimmers.

Goggles

As with a wetsuit, find your best fit! Goggles should feel secure, as you do not want them falling off or filling up with water.

Unfortunately, goggles will fog up, no matter what. Antifog drops, wipes, and sprays tend to work well. An additional option is to soak your goggles in baby shampoo. Place a small amount in the goggle, rinse lightly, and air dry. If you are midswim and need clarity, turn over onto your back, tuck your arms in close like an otter, and clear your goggles with your thumbs.

Always carry a spare pair in your bag for race day.

Swim Aids

Safer Swimmer buoys are a great investment for training, as they provide visibility in the open water. Other swim aids, such as fins, hand paddles, and pull buoys, are valuable pool training tools; however, they are not approved for use in triathlons.

Swim Starts and Entries

You will experience different starting methods during your triathlon career. Race organizers will determine the specific approach based on the number of participants, course, and environment. Here are a few types of starts:

Pool Start (Pool Swim)

As Meredith mentions earlier (see page 32), a pool swim triathlon is a great place to start for a beginner. Usually these are organized as "snake swims," with each swimmer starting several seconds behind the next. Each swimmer "snakes" down the pool by starting in one lane and swimming the length, going under the lane rope, and back in the next lane, providing the total meters of the designated swim.

Wave Starts: This is the most common type of race start. Predetermined groups, usually based on age group and gender, leave about 3 to 5 minutes apart.

Mass Starts: All participants begin at the same time.

Time Trial Starts: Participants line up and begin about 2 to 5 seconds apart.

Pontoon Starts: Participants push off or dive from a pontoon or dock at predetermined intervals.

Positioning Your Start

Choose a starting position based on your comfort level. If you are confident, position yourself out front or at a strategic location to effectively target the first buoy. If you are feeling nervous or would prefer to avoid "traffic," begin near the outer side or back of the pack. Take your time entering the water. The extra 10 to 15 seconds to ease into the start will lend to a more comfortable experience.

Entries will vary for each race. Here are some tips on different types of entries:

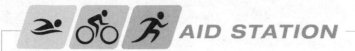
AID STATION

MY FIRST WETSUIT

Meredith here. I knew the day would come: wetsuit day. The Expert and the kids were watching *Jumanji*, while I browsed wetsuits online. Out of the blue, I piped up. "I need a wetsuit," I said.

The Expert looked at me.

He looked at me and laughed. "You know," he said, "that's something I never thought I'd hear come out of your mouth. 'I think I'm going to need a wetsuit.'"

"I imagine it won't be the last weird thing I say doing this triathlon thing," I said.

I thought to myself: *My legs are going to fall off* and *Are there sharks in this water?* were probably also things I would say in the future.

I realized that I could not shop for a wetsuit online. I had no clue what to get. I was told to get *fitted* for the wetsuit. *Oh, the horror. Someone to fit me? Into a wetsuit? What did that mean? Would I have to get naked?*

Regardless, I was not getting out of the wetsuit ordeal. If I wanted to do an open water swim, then I needed a wetsuit to practice swimming in the frigid open water at the nearby lake. (Said nearby lake was a lovely sixty-one degrees, which, in case you were wondering, feels like ice.)

I was feeling helpless and ridiculous. The wetsuit was the part of triathlon that felt most cruel. Me in neoprene? Ugh.

On The Day, my worst fear was realized.

If a wetsuit fits properly, then it will be tight as all hell and require mad skills to properly put it on. Truer words have never been uttered. Wetsuits are like the most evil type of Spanx imaginable.

I walked into the triathlon store very scared. A superfit saleswoman looked at me suspiciously when I asked her about trying on a wetsuit. She eyed my pants.

"Did you bring anything to change into?" she asked me.

"Yep, yep yep, got it right here in my purse." She did not look convinced.

The sizing chart for the women's suit said to add 10 pounds to your *normal* weight and find *that* weight on the chart. Wherever you fell, there

continues

continued

was your wetsuit size. Well, it wasn't *adding* 10 pounds that sent me into the men's sizing chart. Perhaps if the chart said: add 50 pounds.

"Height? Weight?" she asked. *Now is not the time to pull the 20-pound lie. I need this suit to actually fit*, I told myself. So, I took a deep breath and mumbled the numbers. She disappeared for the span of a lifetime and returned with a suit. The suit was shiny and pretty. And had O-R-C-A spelled across the chest.

"Super. Orca?" I whined.

"Orca is a great suit," she said.

"Yeah, for someone like you, Miss Teeny," I said, huffing. Secretly, I was glad to be helped by a female (albeit one with zero body fat). I could just imagine Mr. Male Triathlete wrestling my body into a suit, not knowing what to do with all my extra . . . stuff.

So, Miss Teeny walked me through the ins and outs of wetsuit handling, from turning it inside out and pulling from the inside of the suit only to avoid tearing the neoprene. The whole thing was amazingly difficult. I stopped and had a bit of an out-of-body experience, hovering over myself, as I tend to do quite often. I watched myself struggling into this suit and the whole thing was ridiculous. *I could be at the Olive Garden having all-you-can-eat salad and breadsticks right now! What am I doing here?*

My fingers started cramping before I had the suit over my hips. Miss Teeny helped me pull it up on my arms. This is why it's a good idea to have a buddy help with the wetsuit (you shouldn't be swimming alone, anyway!).

A grand total of forty-five minutes later, I was zipped up and Orca proud. I shook my head as I looked in the mirror, thankful that triathlon is not a beauty pageant.

After the initial shock of the wetsuit applying process, Miss Teeny told me the secret: L-U-B-E. A can of spray lube safe for the wetsuit (I like TriSlide). We were not allowed to use it because, obviously, I had not purchased the suit. But she told me to lather that stuff all over my body (ankles, wrist, arms, legs, everywhere) then, the suit would slide on a million times easier. I was glad to hear it, because if the wetsuit process was that bad all the time, I would be forced to give up my triathlon dreams.

continues

continued

> I walked out with the men's version of the Orca brand suit. Orca. A whale suit. A freaking *Free Willy* suit. *For the love.*
>
> But the mission was accomplished and something about the wetsuit made my Main Goal feel very *real*. Carrying the wetsuit out to the car, it all felt legit. Triathlon and all.

Shore Entry

It is highly recommended to practice entering the surf before you race. Walk the shoreline and entry to determine what the bottom is made of (e.g., sand, rocks, silt, mud, etc,), as well as depth. Practice walking or running into the water. Use a high marching step or high-knee stride. The general rule is to start swimming when the water level hits just above the knee. If you choose to dive forward at this point, make sure you note the depth during your "prewalk" to safely dive in without injury. A shallow dive is always recommended. Be aware of sandbars or other obstructions to avoid while entering the water. Starts in wavy conditions may require the most coordination. Seek guidance from an experienced professional to effectively learn how get under or through a wave.

Deep Water Start

For a deep water start, you may need to float or tread water for a period of time before the race begins. Try to relax and don't kick like crazy. When the starting horn blows, do a strong scissor kick to propel yourself forward and begin freestyle.

Boat Jump

Swimmers line up and jump into the water at frequent intervals. Jump feet first when instructed by race organizers and quickly swim away from the boat. To avoid losing your goggles, hold them in your hand or to your head when hitting the water. Adjust your goggles once you are safely away from the boat and other jumping swimmers.

Ready for Race Day

Upon check-in or packet pickup, you will likely be given a specific color swim cap that corresponds with your start wave, age group, or gender. In most races, you will also get a timing chip associated with your race number. The timing chip will track your swim, bike, run, transitions, and total race time. Find out when the race briefing will take place, as the information given by the race organizers is for your safety and benefit. Proceed to the transition area for setup and preparation.

Warming up on race day can vary based on the individual. Some athletes prefer to do a short swim, if the race allows. Others will stretch, while some may go for a short jog or ride to give their body time to loosen up and get the blood flowing. Find out what works best for you during training.

Walk to where you can see the swim course and buoys, the Swim OUT (where the race starts), Swim IN (where you exit the swim), and pathway to the transition area. Assess the water conditions. If you have time and conditions allow, practice your entry, review the course, and ask yourself:

- Where are the buoys and key turns?
- What will you sight on?
- Do you need to change your breathing pattern based on conditions?

During your swim, remember to stay positive and take it one step and stroke at a time. Focus from buoy to buoy on one topic or technique you've been working on. This will help break down the length of the entire swim into accomplishable sections. Remember to sight early and often to ensure you are on course. There is no need to swim farther than necessary!

Some experts say that training is 90 percent physical and 10 percent mental. When it is time to race, 90 percent of performance becomes mental. Stay positive during your swim. Repeat your swim mantras, such as "Just keep swimming," "Breathe and relax," or whatever suits you best.

Sing a song like "Amazing Grace" or even "Happy Birthday" (anything with a calming rhythm) might help. You can also count your strokes, or think of a particular person for whom you might like to dedicate your swim.

Remember your safety stroke and rely on it as needed. Note where safety vessels are located before and during your swim. If you need assistance, wave your hand in the air to gain the attention of a first responder or volunteer. You are allowed to rest on a kayak, rescue tube, or noodle, as long as you do not make forward progress. Take your time and catch your breath.

As you approach the swim exit, about one length of the pool away, slightly increase your kick to generate blood flow to the legs. This will help prepare you for the run to transition when exiting the swim. Get excited that you have successfully completed the swim—the first leg of your triathlon! Hooray!

7 THE BIKE

A S A YOUNG CHILD, I WAS UNABLE TO *STOP* MY BIKE. THE neighborhood trash cans all bore marks from my running bull-in-a-China-shop-style into them. I would go and go on the bike, and if I needed to stop, I would simply barrel into the nearest plastic curbside can. To this day, the biggest challenge for me is stopping and getting off my bike in one piece.

--- NEW RIDER TIP ---

Always use the same foot to start and stop pedaling, and the same foot to put down when you stop. This will help you gain confidence with your stops and starts, especially when you begin to work with clipless pedals.

After making my Decision to become a triathlete, I was determined to get moving right away. I dusted off my old road bike and wheeled it out of the garage. *I was going to be a triathlete! I needed to ride a bike! I was going to ride a bike! Here I go!*

My bike was a bright yellow Giant OCR3, ancient as all hell, but with only 50 miles of actual wear on it.

On the first day of my determined bicycle riding, I packed G-Force (the bike) into the car and bade the Expert farewell. The Expert just stared at me with his mouth open as I pulled out of the driveway.

The Expert loved to ride his bike and he had ridden for many years. In fact, I gave him a hard time about spending time *away* from me and loving his bike more, which was a great point of contention in our early marriage. So, eight years later, I was fairly certain that as I pulled out of the driveway, he was probably saying out loud, "Oh, sure, *now* she wants to ride a bike. All those years she kept *me* from riding, but now . . . oh boy . . . "

I returned home only a short time later.

The Expert was not surprised. He was kind of smirking, actually. I walked in the door, slammed my keys on the counter, and said two words.

"I quit."

"How can you quit? You just started." Eye roll from him.

"I don't want to talk about it," I said.

Okay, so I was not *really* going to quit. But quitting crossed my mind during that first bike ride. What was so terrible about that first ride? For starters, about a half mile into the maiden voyage, I hit a big hill. I did not know what to do with my bike on a hill. I thought I had downshifted, but actually I was grinding out the hill in my giant gear, all the while thinking, *You have to be effing kidding me! This is cycling? Horrible!*

Then, I began to feel as though I would pass out. My legs were also fighting against me and I began to roll backward down the hill. Determined not to roll backward, I teetered and cursed and instead, I fell sideways. *Riding a bike is miserable!* I rode for another twenty minutes, searching for small hills that I could navigate. But I hated every last second of it. Despite the fact I only rode about 5 miles, I drove home completely wiped out and defeated.

As I told the Expert my tale, I dragged him over to the bike and pointed my blaming finger at G-Force, declaring that the stupid, ugly, old bike was broken.

The Expert pointed to the shifter, "This is broken?"

I glared at him. But being the lawyer I was, I decided I would entertain his argument.

"How do you shift when you get on a hill?" he asked me.

I showed him, by gesturing.

"Umm-hmmmmm," he muttered. "And how do you shift when you go down a hill?"

I showed him again.

"Nope. Wrong!"

The Expert assured me that I would have a much more enjoyable time once I learned *how* to use my bike. He said I just had no earthly idea how to shift.

"When you see a big hill coming, you need to put it in the Granny Grocery Getter Gear," he said.

"The what?"

"*Ring ring!* The groceries are here!"

I looked at him.

"Like a granny bike. Like a slow granny riding a bike with a basketful of groceries. With a bell. *Ring ring!*"

I stared at him.

He laughed, "You want to be in an 'easy' gear, like you are taking a casual trip to the grocery store. You want easy because that results in the biggest chance of succeeding up the hill and not blowing up your legs."

Recognition. I smiled.

"You were simply in the buster gear."

"Buster?"

"Yeah. Ball buster," the Expert said.

I may have been ready to become a triathlete in my dreams, but I was not ready for actually riding a bike. In retrospect, I wanted to quit because

I was not *prepared* for riding. I had not learned how to shift gears, to corner. I had failed to learn the basics that actually make riding *enjoyable*.

The next few times I went to ride with G-Force, things *still* did not go so well for me. I crashed. Twice. I do not mean real heroic or cool crashes. I mean superlame crashes.

But—due to stubbornness—eventually, I had a good bike ride. And part of the good ride was finding a beautiful new bike that was fitted for *me*. I named her "Antonia" and she became my new bike companion.

I was nice to her. I learned how to clip into her pedals, to clip out and dismount safely. I learned to clean her up, make her shiny, change her tire tubes, inflate her tires, and fix her dropped chain. Eventually, I did not run into parked cars and trash cans. Cycling started out as my biggest enemy, but quickly became the sport in triathlon I enjoy the most.

Over the course of the last almost-decade, I have had four new-to-me bikes, including three triathlon bikes (which we will discuss later). Each bike does, indeed, have its own personality, fit, and flair. As in any relationship, we must keep working at the bike until it works for us—not against us. Sometimes there is simply not any chemistry with a certain bike or the fit is logistically bad. Take heart—your bike love will come—you just need to search for them and make them yours.

THE BIKE ITSELF

One must have a bike to do triathlon. One need not, however, have an expensive and fancy bike. Just *a* bike. You can do a sprint triathlon on *any* bike. Technically, you can do most any triathlon on any bike (within the rules of the race). If you want to go faster, be more efficient, and race longer distances, you should choose a more efficient bike. However, for your first or next triathlon, you can literally use any bike—even ole Rusty in your garage—provided you attend to a few things.

If you use ole Rusty, then he needs to: fit you reasonably well *and* be safe for yourself and those around you. Other than that? There are not many other requirements. So, congratulations, you have a bike!

My favorite local bike shop, Cannon Cyclery in Atlanta, owned by Curtis Henry, has done amazing things to teach me about my two-wheels. Because proper cycling form, racing, and more begin with a proper bike fit, comfort, and alignment, I asked Curtis to share his expertise here. With over seventeen years of experience working on everything from kids' bikes to race bikes, there is very little Curtis has not seen. I've heard him called the "Best Wrench in Atlanta" more times than you'd think possible. That's a compliment, by the way.

ABOUT THE BIKE

Curtis Henry
Cannon Cyclery, Atlanta
www.cannoncyclery.bike

Types of Bikes

When getting yourself going on a new two-wheeled machine, it's easy to get overwhelmed—overwhelmed with options, or worse, stuck in analysis-paralysis. For the purpose of tri, there are several bikes that will get the job done, but as in most sports, some things are better than others. As mentioned, it's totally possible to complete a tri on any bike (beach cruiser included, although probably not the best idea). No rules specify what type of bike you must use, just that the contraption *is* a bike and has no motor to propel you forward without your own power.

Road Bikes

Road bikes are built to roll on mostly paved surfaces and are generally focused on efficiency and speed. Road bikes feature lightweight frames, drop-style handlebars for a more aerodynamic body position, and speed-oriented wheels and gearing. The handlebar style is made for multiple hand locations, which allows for several riding positions to accommodate both long and shorter distances. "Roadies" are made for climbing and descending roads, carving turns, group riding, and come in many varieties.

Tri Bikes

A triathlon or a time trial bike (we'll call both a "tri bike") is the usual road machine choice for the intermediate to advanced tri geek. A tri bike takes many of the features found on a road bike and incorporates an aerodynamic frame, handlebar, and wheels.

The tri bike is built around a handlebar system called aerobars, which are made for basically a lying position supported by your elbows. The position is usually aggressive and is made to be aerodynamic—so I would use caution as a beginner using this type of bike. Give racing a season or two with a road bike if you are new to cycling, before diving into a tri bike.

Mountain Bikes and Hybrids

Mountain bikes, designed for unpaved surfaces, have some specific features that make them especially useful for riding on dirt, gravel, rocks, and the nasty off-road stuff that you encounter on a trail or gravel road.

Hybrids are a mash-up of specific features that strive to be do-it-all machines. Generally, a hybrid combines the quick rolling wheels of a road bike with the gearing and flat handlebar of a mountain bike. They have more upright riding positions and are built around ride comfort and versatility. They work well for things like commuting, family riding, neighborhood riding, etc.

Deals on Bikes

Plenty of resources are available online to help get a bike search going, but your local bike shop (LBS) will be your best resource. It will be there to support you and take care of your new machine, so get to know the staff and try to glean some advice.

Budget

Come up with a budget for a new bike that is realistic for you and your goals. And stick to it. Bear in mind that a cheap bike is usually just that:

a cheap ride quality and plenty of nagging mechanical issues. The quality of the bike has a lot to do with the quality of the experience.

If you are involved in a tri or cycling club, take advantage of the discounts that are often available to you.

Used and Closeouts

Gently used is a great way to start, especially when it comes from a shop that has serviced and checked the bike over. Used bikes from a good shop will be clean, tuned, and ready to go. The selection is often quite varied, but if you happen to find something that fits your size and budget, it can be a sweet hookup. The trade-off when going used is a lack of warranty. The factory warranty on a bike only applies to the original owner, so make sure to do your homework and check for any recalls, common failures, or bad press. If you're feeling brave, venture out to the used market; just be sure you're educated and invest the time into the process. Going used can be good but can come with some risk as well.

Closeouts and last year's models are a great way to get something new for a sweet deal. Most brands will dump their remaining inventory to dealers, wholesalers, and online retailers, so if you know what you're looking for (from your research), you can often find a fantastic deal. Just because it's not the latest and greatest model does not mean it's not a great bike. The bike retail market is changing and it's rare to find exactly what you want in stock these days, so don't be afraid to ask your shop to look for a closeout model or something from last season.

Avoid the Department Store

Although tempting when you're dipping your toe into the world of cycling and triathlon, a department store bike will come back to haunt you every time. Whether it's ongoing mechanical issues, uncomfortable seat and fit, heavy sluggish ride, or general poor ride quality, you will not enjoy the riding experience. Department store bikes are, for the most part, big kids' bikes that are okay for kids—but often not best for adults. That being said, if you have a department store bike and want to use it for your first triathlon—try and take it to your LBS to get it in the best shape possible.

Hear the Right Voices

Remember to go with the experts and experienced people in your life when listening to recommendations. Start local and do your best to support the local economy with your purchases. Look for shops that have a consignment program or trade in program.

Intangibles

Do you love a particular color, style, or brand? Remember that this part is secondary to the rest. However, when forming a relationship with your bike, it's important to love it! So, find a happy medium on fit and fabulous.

Bike Components

Your drivetrain (chain, gears, derailleurs, shifters, and crank/pedals) works together to turn your leg motion into wheel motion; which is an important job on a bicycle! Because this is *the* entire point of a bicycle, it's vitally important to know what a good drivetrain (and a bad one!) is. For the most part, the quality of the drivetrain parts is in line with the amount of money you spend. As you spend more, you get lighter weight, better-shifting quality, as well as longer-lasting parts that stay in adjustment properly.

Ultimately, you'll want to go for something simple and easy to use— not the cheapest but also *not* the most expensive. That way you will have a pleasant experience getting acquainted with your bike without having to deal with drivetrain issues.

Bike Fit

Finding a good bike fitter and getting your new bike properly fitted is a crucial step with a new bike. This process can help you get properly set up on the bike as well as make sure you're using the bike to its potential while avoiding injuries. A bike that is properly fitted to your individual needs and goals is the best way to achieve maximum efficiency, comfort, and power on your wheeled rocket.

You need a hands-on approach to make sure the fit is done right, but many tools are available to help the process. Have a quick interview with a few bike fit specialists and find someone who has experience with the type of bike you want, as some fitters have more experience in one type than another.

A comprehensive bike-fitting process covers everything from pedals to shifters. A good fitter should work through your athletic and injury history along with an interview to figure out how you got here and where you are going with the bike.

During the process, several things can be adjusted and should be measured. The process should generally start with your cleats and move forward to your hands. The following should be analyzed: seat height and position, knee angle, knee position, hip position, hip and torso angles, reach to the handlebars/aerobars, as well as weight distribution.

Most of all, enjoy your new ride!

TIME TO RIDE (LIKE, FOR REAL)

Meredith here. Okay, so we now have a properly-fitted-for-you bicycle. We have a shiny new helmet and water bottles. Now what? Do you just get on your bike and Forrest Gump to nowhere—bicycle version? You *could*, but let's not and say we did.

So, where in the world *should* you ride?

Always remember to put safety first. Riding in traffic is daunting even for experienced cyclists, because we are at the mercy of drivers on the road. No matter how careful we may be, *other* drivers and cyclists may not be as careful. Not to scare you away, but do your best to find a safe path, especially in the beginning.

You have a few options for riding your bike—who knew there were so many creative ways to ride a bike? Yay, technology! Here are our options: indoor bike trainer, indoor cycling classes, neighborhood riding, mountain bike trails, closed-paved trail riding, and then hitting the road-road (and also group riding).

Indoor Bike Trainer

The indoor bike trainer is an amazing tool for building bike fitness, learning to improve your cadence, technique, and strength. A bike *trainer* is *not* a human being who yells at you like a boot camp sergeant. Rather, a trainer is an indoor mechanism that allows you to ride your bike indoors.

Without going into nauseating detail, you can basically attach your bike upright to the trainer by using the rear wheel skewer, or by removing the wheel and affixing the rear frame of the bike to the trainer. Once it is in place, you then can ride *your* bike just like a much-harder-to-pedal stationary bike. You can find a good trainer for a couple hundred bucks, or you can invest your savings in one. You are safe indoors and can binge-watch your favorite shows. Technology has come such a long way, too (and will continue), in that you can ride courses on your smart trainer and race other riders on your phone or laptop. If you intend to train and do triathlons, a bike trainer is a necessary tool. However, it's not paramount to getting to your *first* triathlon.

Bike trainers *are* important if you live in severe climates—especially if you experience snow and ice into the late spring. The trainer is also good for rainy days. Eventually, you might decide to tackle some rainy-day rides. However, riding in the rain takes some experience and you should put your health and well-being first. In rain, snow, sleet, and hail, the trainer allows you to ride and watch television at the same time!

The benefits of working out on a bike trainer are many. Because you must keep a consistent force on the pedals (or the pedals will stop spinning), it is rumored in the bike community that two hours on the trainer is like putting in three hours on the bike outside. Additionally, you can use the bike trainer to work your cycling drills (more on this follows).

Indoor Cycling Classes

Indoor cycling classes at a gym or triathlon club are a great foundation for cycling outdoors. These classes are a good place to practice your form and cadence, as well as increase overall fitness. However, "riding a bike to nowhere" is a different experience than feeling the wind on your face and actually moving down a road. Therefore, while training in cycling class is definitely beneficial, especially in the colder months, you must get yourself out on the road and on your bike before triathlon-ing.

In cycling class, the bikes are often the Spinner brand bikes, but there are many, many different brands of indoor cycling bikes. Additionally, some places host indoor trainer rides where you bring your trainer and bike for group fun. Of course, now with technology there are at-home cycling bikes with large screens where you can ride virtually with an instructor, too. These are all great options.

Neighborhood Riding

This may seem like a weird section, but if you live in a neighborhood that's light on traffic, then taking off on a few loops around the hood is not a bad idea. Sure, you may think: *My neighbors will see me!* But I have some news for you—eventually everyone will see you, so get used to it. This is easy, also, for when you start to ride longer—getting accustomed to the routes leaving straight from your driveway are big time savers. Additionally, if you have young children, this is a way to get in some extra miles and family time. Just keep your expectations low: you won't be doing any hard-core training circling your neighborhood and cul-de-sac; however, this might be a good start for many of us.

Mountain Bike Trails

I won't cover mountain biking because it's a book unto itself. However, if you have a mountain bike, this is an option for getting those miles in. A reminder, too, that you *can* totally do your first triathlon on a mountain bike. While it's not perfection for a tri, it *will* work.

Closed-Paved Trails

I recommend paved trails for beginner cyclists, but with a long list of caveats. Because these routes are closed to motorized traffic, they seem to be the safest option around, and arguably they are—pedestrians and dogs are certainly less dangerous than tractor trailers. At the same time, hazards are hazards. Walkers, runners, strollers, Rollerbladers, and cyclists are allowed on these trails—and we are all hazards for each other.

Bear in mind that you may need to drive 10 or 20 miles outside of town to find a safe place to ride. Invest in a bike rack for your car and *go*. The safety factor is worth the investment. Constantly fearing cars and traffic lights will put a damper on any ride.

Remember to be aware of your surroundings on a trail. Not everyone will be a great student of safety like you have become—and they may not know what "on your left" means. And if you see dogs without leashes? Run. Er, pedal away—fast.

Road Riding

I do not recommend cycling on the road with traffic until several thresholds are met. While getting on the road as early as possible is a goal, safety and confidence must take precedence.

Before you hit the road with traffic, you should be able to: ride 8 to 10 miles comfortably, stop your bike and dismount at a moment's notice, have the ability to "hold your line" (i.e., ride in a straight line), understand road safety and hand signals, check/glance behind you while keeping your bike straight, and not be deathly afraid of the road.

Sounds like you will never get there? You will. Now, it doesn't mean that all these things need to be perfect, but you should have the vast majority under control before venturing on the road with traffic. Start with the neighborhood. Ride to a light, dismount, stop, hand signal—lather, rinse, repeat. Baby steps.

Call your local bike shop and ask where you can find a good, yet safe (relatively low-car-traffic) ride. You can also spend some time with Google and ask it where some fabulous routes are located. Additionally, the Internet and social media is a great place to flesh out rides. Many cyclists post their favorite riding routes via certain websites, and you can download their hardworking route(s) and see whether their favorite places are a good fit for you in terms of both location and distance.

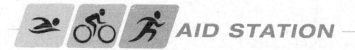 **AID STATION**

A DOG TIP

Sometimes when riding a vicious stray dog will start to chase you. I have found the best thing to do is to try to stay on your path and ride away. Focus on the road, not the dog. If you are comfortable riding one-handed, spray the dog with your water bottle—this is usually sufficient to confuse and deter it. Some riders carry pepper spray for this reason, but I won't be a proponent of spraying animals with pepper spray. At the same time, it's your life so protect yourself how you see fit. Just do whatever it takes not to hit the dog (you'll go flying!) or get tangled up with a dog (you'll get bitten *and* possibly go flying).

Group Riding

Group riding is a surprisingly good idea for beginners, although it seems terrifying. Again, this is for beginners who have crossed over to some comfort and experience on their bikes. While riding in a group will be scary at first, it is something that must be conquered if you ride regularly and race. Go with a good friend, and find a "no drop" ride. *No drop* means that *no* cyclist (even you!) will be left behind.

From a safety standpoint, riding with more than one cyclist is preferable, for the sake of visibility. But just as for cars, you also need to watch out for your fellow riders.

AT THE END of the day, wherever or however you ride, be aware of your equipment and surroundings. I know many people who have fallen off Spin bikes and bike trainers. So that, too, is possible. If outside, always remember to be aware of your surroundings and be cautious. If in doubt, stop, look, and listen.

There is no substitute for time actually spent on the bike. Simple put, the more you ride, the better you will become; the more comfortable you will be; and the more fun you will have.

SAVE YOUR QUEEN (AND I'M NOT TALKING CHESS)

Extended periods in the bike saddle are hard on your rear end. When I say your rear end, I mean your buns *and* your lady parts: aka "the Queen." Plain and simple, the Queen will start to scream after so many miles. The best way to deal with this issue? Ride more. Seriously. The Queen is a lazy diva who must be whipped into shape, and only time in the saddle will save her! God save the Queen!

That being said, be nice to the Queen. Get her a good saddle, proper bike fit, comfy chamois (padded) shorts, and lots of lubricant to keep her happy. If you are noticing that the Queen goes completely numb while you are riding, then you are ripe for a noseless saddle. Basically, these seats remove the pointy part of the saddle, which in turn takes the pressure off the Queen and her castle. Although the Expert does not have a Queen, he uses one of these saddles, too, and says it helps with the Jesters (you don't need me to spell that out, do you?). As I upped my distances, I changed saddles once again.

In the beginning, you may need a padded seat cover. But please, I beg you, do not rely on this. With a proper bike fit, you should not need the extreme padding (which will also interfere with the efficiency of your pedal stroke). Plus, you want to get the Queen in shape, remember!

Sometimes you can develop "saddle sores." Saddles sores are skin issues on the Queen or her backyard neighbors, the Humps. Saddle sores can appear from too much unnecessary chafing and movement (forward, backward, side to side) in the bike saddle—which is precisely why a good bike fit is paramount. If you are too high in the saddle, your body and hips will move too much and you are ripe for sores.

Also, keep the Queen clean and lubed up and wear a one-piece chamois pad while in the saddle. A chamois pad can be made with two or more pieces, causing additional friction and discomfort.

And while it may be entirely too much information, I personally feel that the Queen is a better cycling partner when she is completely bald. Less chance for ingrown you-know-whats and ripped-out-you-know-whats. Others may disagree, so just allow the Queen to coif her style however she'd like. She is, after all, the Queen.

HOW TO RIDE YOUR BIKE

As a beginner triathlete, I was scared to death of riding my bike: flat roads, hills, traffic   it did not matter—all of it was horrifying. I slowly became accustomed to riding on a paved, flat trail. But I continued to remain terrified of climbing hills.

The bike was not the problem. The problem was not the size of the hill, because I would run from *all* hills. The problem was *me*. I had not learned to ride efficiently, and it made me scared to climb.

Arguably, riding your bike has less to do with the actual bike than you might think. If you have a decent bike, then really, the rest is up to the *rider*. Cycling, like swimming, is much about technique, form, and a little bit of coordination. To be an efficient cyclist, there are rules of the road and ways to do (and not to do) the second sport of triathlon.

Heart Rate Training for the Bike

Heart rate training is outlined in detail in the Run section (pages 133–149). Outside of intense testing that might be confusing at this juncture, for simplicity's sake, your bike heart rate zones tend to be ten beats per minute *lower* than your personal running zones. So, if you can test your running heart rate zones, you can guesstimate your cycling zones.

For a more accurate reading of your cycling heart rate zones, you can perform what is known as the lactate threshold test. I like to use Joe Friel's version for my athletes, which can be executed and summarized as this.[1]

"To find your LTHR, do a 30-minute time trial all by yourself (no training partners and not in a race). Again, it should be done *as if it was a race for the entire 30 minutes*. But at 10 minutes into the test, click the lap button on your heart rate monitor. When done, look to see what your average heart rate was for the last 20 minutes. That number is an approximation of your LTHR.

"I am frequently asked if you should go hard for the first 10 minutes. The answer is, 'Yes, go hard for the entire 30 minutes.' But be aware that most people doing this test go too hard the first few minutes and then gradually slow down for the remainder. That will give you inaccurate results. The more times you do this test the more accurate your LTHR is likely to become as you will learn to pace yourself better at the start."[2]

If you have an electronic training log specifically for endurance athletes (such as TrainingPeaks), you can then enter this data into the program and it will help figure these numbers for you. However, if you are not able to use something, then you can use these calculations.

Bike Zones
Zone 1 Less than 81% of LTHR
Zone 2 81% to 89% of LTHR
Zone 3 90% to 93% of LTHR
Zone 4 94% to 99% of LTHR
Zone 5 100% to 106% of LTHR
(There are also Zones 5a, 5b, and 5c, which can be further used for training and testing.)

Make Sure You Are Ready to Ride

This goes back to your bike fit, bike bag, confidence, knowledge of the road rules, and all your gear. Take the bike for a few test rides around the block to make sure that everything feels right. Practice shifting gears a few times. Sometimes the ride around the block will save you a lot of trouble on the road.

"Purposeful Suffering"

Gerry is fond of the phrase "purposeful suffering." In other words, we are embarking on training days to suffer—on purpose! He swears by "making friends" with the pain, the hills, and the hard rides. You set out to suffer with a purpose. You suffer. And suffer. And through the suffering, you make the improvements happen.

A great tip from Gerry is: "Acknowledge that the suffering is about to commence. You should prepare your mind to focus on the effort. Embrace the purposeful suffering. Make best friends with the pain. Love it."

Because the truth is—sometimes riding is hard and just sucks.

Where Can You Relax?

I bet you are thinking, *I can relax back on my couch at home. Or on a beach in the Bahamas.*

But "Where can you relax?" is a great question to ask to remind yourself to keep your body in a calm and relaxed state when riding. This means keeping your elbows relaxed and your shoulders down. Keeping your upper body completely relaxed—right down to your face muscles— saves energy and makes the bike ride easier.

Do not lock your elbows. Do not clench your hands to the point of white knuckles. Do not scrunch your face. Do not grind your teeth. Keep everything up top relaxed and you will be amazed at the energy it saves on the bottom (and the next day!). I was not naturally able to relax. (What a surprise.) But now, I practice relaxation everywhere, including in cycling class and when I am in the car in Atlanta traffic.

As you are going uphill, keep your chest open, with your elbows close to your body and kinda loosey-goosey. When you are riding, ask yourself the simple question "Where can I relax?" You likely are tensing something, and this will be a good reminder to find the place of tension, release it, and save energy.

This small tip (of course, from Gerry) makes a massive difference.

Learn Your Gears

Whether you are riding on flat land or in the hills, you must find the right gear(s) for your terrain. Look, gearing takes practice. Period. Take your bike on rides and practice, practice, practice.

Let's let our bike guy Curtis explain: "Every bike shifting system is slightly different, but are all designed to basically do one thing: make your cadence consistent. When your pedaling cadence is coupled with the right gearing you get mechanical advantage over the terrain. Therefore, learning and understanding what cadence to pedal at will help this process.

"Spend some time getting to know how your shifters work and get comfortable with them. For the most part, shifters are intuitive—they have levers and triggers that push and release the chain up and down the cassette and chainrings.

"Some use two levers, some use one, and the electronic systems use buttons, but they all move the chain up and down your gears. So, get to know what lever does what, and as you spend more time on the bike, it will become second nature. Once you have mastered the function of your shifting system, it's time to work on the cadence thing.

"The goal is to use the gears in different combinations to maintain a consistent cadence. The gearing is designed to give you mechanical advantage up, down, and on flat surfaces for varied speeds, but the trick is to keep your cadence consistent. So, if you are trying to maintain a 75 rpm with your feet, try to stay within 10 rpm of that while shifting up and down the gearing over the terrain you're riding on.

"One of the other things that may help you remember how and when to shift is to think about the gearing in terms of ranges instead of numbers. Try to think about your bicycle's chain as a straight line and its position relative to the centerline of the bike. As the chain gets closer to the centerline of the bike, the gearing gets easier for more mechanical advantage or a lower range, and when it's farther away, the gearing gets harder for more speed in a higher range. Regardless of what brand of components and shifters you have, this trick works for every bike with traditional derailleurs. Just remember when the chain goes farther away from the center of the bike, to the right, the gearing will get harder and easier to the left. Boom, easy!"

(Thanks, Curtis!)

Hill riding is especially challenging for a beginner because of the intricacies of learning to gear. When you see a hill on the horizon, do not turn around and go the other way—as I used to do. You must learn to enjoy the hills, and part of learning to love them is learning how to ride them.

Most standard road and triathlon bikes will have two front rings: large and small. The large gear will serve you well on downhills and flat roads; the small gear is for climbing, heading out of transition and general starting after stopping. (Tip: It is easier to "go" in an easy gear. When you are approaching a stop light or sign, you can shift into lower gears to make the restart easier.)

You want to get in the easiest, lower gears to climb a reasonably steep hill—meaning you want your bike to be in the smaller front chain ring. However, do not slam the bike into the lowest gear when you see a hill coming. That will make a mess and cause you to overspin, possibly topple over, and make a fool out of yourself.

(I am not sure how I know this. I plead the Fifth.)

Finding the right gear for each particular hill takes practice, but eventually you will instinctively know where you need to be gear-wise. I find that, with the larger climbs, it helps to make a move with your gears *before* you are on the mean, nasty hill and being devoured by it. As a rule of thumb, you do not want to be pushing too hard uphill (grinding in the big chainring, blowing up your leg muscles and knees by struggling to turn the pedals)—nor should you be spinning out of control (slipping into the small ring too early, pedaling wildly and bouncing all over the place). All of this takes practice.

If you can buzz up a short hill quickly and it will not blow up your legs, then do not waste your time fooling with the gears and just pop over the hill. If you grossly underestimated the hill, and when you are halfway up you realize you are about to be in fall-over-type-trouble—you may want to pop out of the saddle and get over the hill that way.

─────── POP OUT OF THE SADDLE? WHAT? ───────

Sometimes it may be easier to stand and pedal to get over short hills. This is known as "popping out of the saddle." Sounds like splitting your pants, but it's not. Think: Tour de France.

This takes a little practice and should be used sparingly because it can take a toll on your legs on a long ride.

Your bike should be fitted with the proper cassette for easier (read: beginner) gearing. Make sure you ask your local bike shop for a beginner cassette (or an 11/28 is a good starting point), so you have many options and easy gears to help you over the hills. Nothing will ruin your day faster than "professional" equipment and a giant hill. (I have learned this. Also. The. Hard. Way.)

Push Your Butt Back!

When you see a hill coming, stay seated and push your rear end toward the rear of the saddle. Be careful not to push your butt *off* the back of the saddle.

Why? Well, as you drive your feet downward on the downstroke, you will be engaging your quads (front leg muscles) and glutes (your bun muscles) to push forward. When your butt is back, you are in a position of greater power. Also, remember to lean your upper body ever so slightly forward to keep your center of gravity in . . . well, the center.

Repeat Song Lyrics

Another cycling tip is to repeat rap lyrics when the ride gets difficult. Okay, so this is a silly tip. But somehow repeating the rhythmic lyrics to "'Till I Collapse" in my head gets me up any hill much faster.

Eyes and Head UP

When you are riding, keep your head up, eyes wide, and chest open. Do not look at the ground. Do not look down at your bike. Keep your head up to allow your airways to remain open and get oxygen to those punished lungs. Not to mention, you really should be looking ahead at the road at all times.

Keeping your eyes on the road does not mean looking on the road directly in front of you. Just as if you were driving a car, you should look *down* the road, so you can take in all the dangers, conditions, and scenery.

At the same time, you still want to glance directly in front of you to make sure there are no potholes or gravel in the road. I tend to scan my eyes farther down the road every so often to ensure the road conditions are good, so I have time to avoid bad pavement or shenanigans if necessary.

Downhills and Braking

Riding a bike *is* dangerous, more dangerous than many of us realize. Some good tips I have received from the Expert (who is actually a very good technical cyclist and mountain biker) and others: err on the side of caution and slower speeds, especially on a downhill.

Even if you are flying downhill like a bat out of cycling hell, do *not* suddenly grab your brakes or squeeze them too hard. An important tip is to *ease* into braking. When you are headed downhill, your body's center of gravity is toward the front wheel. Do your best to keep your butt back on the seat as much as you can to keep your center of gravity *away* from the front.

Brake carefully, lightly, and steadily to control your speed on a down-hill. Be careful with your front brakes: if you use excessive front braking you risk going over the handlebars. And by "going over the handlebars," I mean *your body* flying off your bike, *over* the handlebars and *onto* the pavement. (Eeeek.) On bikes sold in the United States, the front brake will typically be the one you squeeze with your left hand. But you can confirm by simply squeezing and looking at your brakes. The one that moves when you squeeze? *Ta-da!*

When you are approaching a turn, slow down and brake *before* you turn the corner. This is the same concept as driving a car. You do not take a corner in a car on two wheels and *then* apply the brakes. You slow down first, then turn. Same principles apply on a bike. Be sure to release the brake levers as you turn. If the front tire hits some loose sand or gravel around a corner *while* you are braking, you can cause the front tire to lock down and the bike to slip out from under you. Learn to ease into braking and use more pressure on your back brake.

A good habit is to rely most heavily on the back brake. I tend to use the front brake *only* when I am cycling in a straight line—such as on a trail. This is more of a habit-forming tip, which will prevent you from using the front break in a sudden or emergency situation. If you stay off the front brake, then you will have less chance of throwing yourself over the handlebars in a panicked moment.

Don't Take the Downhills "Off"

This might feel like a bit of an advanced move, and maybe it is—so take it how you will depending on your experience level. Within the bounds of safety, if you can keep pedaling and working hard *downhill*, you will have a speed advantage over riders who take the downhills "off" so as to rest.

To use this tactic, you need to put your bike in the bigger gears (large front chainring) to get the benefit of the downhill *and* the pedaling. Not only will this give you a time advantage, but you will become a stronger cyclist because—well, you're simply pedaling more.

—— LET'S TALK ABOUT CLIPLESS PEDALS ——

If you decide to get into the sport of triathlon, you will eventually need clipless pedals. Seems like a dumb term, because "clipless" makes you think that you are "without clips." And you are. You are "with cleats"—which are attached to the bottom of your shoes.

Clipless pedals allow your bike shoes to slide into a locking mechanism on your bike pedal. So, yes —once you slide your bike shoe into the pedal, you are essentially attached to your bike—like best friends forever.

Certainly, this might feel terrifying. But as far as fitness, power, speed, and logistics are concerned, this becomes a cycling necessity.

Here's why. If you usual a traditional pedal, you are simply pushing *down* on the pedals—and pushing down *only*. When you are attached to the bike, you are able to maximize and utilize the power of the upstroke (pulling up) and pulling back, in addition to the down stroke.

If you can swing it, just use these from the very beginning. Most pedal systems have a tension system where you can set the tension, making it easier to clip in and out of the pedals—so you can "escape" with ease. If you are new, simply set the tension light and practice on grass, in case of a tumble.

With clipless pedals, you will instantly gain 25 to 40 percent more pedal stroke efficiency (depending on your own efficiency). This is because you are using the *full circular* pedal rotation. In other words, when you are *pushing down* with one leg, you are also *pulling up* with the other.

Perfect Pedal Circles

By using those clipless pedals for what they were designed, you can place power where it matters and become an efficient cyclist. We want to constantly have "smooth pedal strokes."

This means keeping your feet *flat* in the bottom of the pedal stroke, like scraping gum off the bottom of your cycling shoe. If you are riding on your toes or with your toes pointed down, you are engaging the wrong muscles and losing power. A way to tell: do your calves *absolutely* kill you after a cycling workout? You are likely "toe-ing up" and engaging the wrong muscles. Engage your hips on the upstroke to maintain a perfectly engaged, circular pedal stroke, which is a push *and* pull motion.

In other words, use *the entire pedal stroke* to your advantage. Up and down. Up and down. Do not just stomp your feet downward—also remember to pull upward on the pedal.

See? Perfect circles. Like the ones under my eyes.

Keep Your Knees In

"Ride with your knees pushed close together—not touching, of course—but reasonably close. Your knees should be within the distance between your shoulders," my friend Mike Lenhart once said in an interview.

"If you saw a car come down the highway and the two front doors were open, that wouldn't be very efficient (not to mention dangerous). Same deal with riding your bike. Keep the knees in. Otherwise, you're like a circus unicycle rider!" Not only will you look funny, but you will be losing power and risking injury, especially to your knees and hips.

Safety and Group Riding Tips

Wear your helmet. Always.

Wear your sunglasses (yes, this is for eyeball safety!). If it's dark outside, then wear clear ones.

Wear your safety ID.

Do not ride on the sidewalk.

Do not ride with headphones. Seriously. Don't.

Do not talk on your phone (!).

Pretend you are a car. Ride on the same side of the road as the cars, *with* the traffic. For example, in the United States, you will want to ride on the right side of the road.

If you are riding with a group, use signals, such as pointing at the road below to indicate to the riders behind you that there is something in the road (e.g., pothole, crack, debris). This will help the people behind you avoid dangers that you can clearly see.

Use hand signals for turning.

If there is a car coming up from the rear, shout "Car back!" to the riders in front of you to let them know. Same with "Car up!" to signal there is an oncoming car before a turn or stop.

If you are at an intersection and the road is clear to cross, you can shout "Clear!" or "Clear right and clear left!" and proceed to cross. This will signal to the riders behind you that it is safe to cross, so they do not have to clip out of their pedals. Of course, you will want to be certain that it is, in fact, clear. Additionally, make sure that they are just a few seconds behind you, because obviously what seems clear can change pretty quickly.

Learn to "hold your line"– meaning, to ride in a straight line. And stay there.

Look over your left shoulder every once in a while to check for cars, other riders, and so on, but learn to do so without also veering in the direction that you are looking. This takes practice, because our body wants to steer the bike in the direction of our head, so practice this often.

Stay as far right as you possibly and safely can. Note that when the roads are wet, you should stay off of the painted lines, because they are slick when wet.

No "cross wheeling." In other words, don't ride too close behind *and* to the *side* of other riders. If they veer to the right and you are too close behind and to the side, then your front wheel may get caught in their *rear* wheel and cause a crash.

It is fun to ride side by side and chit-chat with your friends. Keep in mind that this is (technically) poor cycling etiquette and annoying to the cars and trucks sharing the road. At the same time, this is part of the fun of group rides. Just bear in mind that if you are on a well-traveled route, you should ride in a single file; save the side-by-side rides for empty country roads.

HOW DO YOU GET FASTER AND BETTER?

"Okay, got it, but I wanna go fast!"

Riding more frequently is the key to becoming a better cyclist. Ideally, riding outside is awesome and will make you more accustomed to the road, force you to learn to terrain ride and climb (if you're in an area with hills). However, if you want to take your cycling up another notch, here are a few beginner tips for next-level notching.

Pay Attention to Your Technique (Like, Really)

As we discussed earlier, your cadence and pedal stroke are very important for riding. Using both the push and pull motion is important to utilize all of the pedal stroke. Relaxing your upper body and engaging your legs and glutes in the pedaling is part of becoming a more efficient cyclist. Simply being mindful when you are on the road of your technique and form will pay large dividends in the long run.

Focus on Cadence

In simplest terms, cadence is the measurement of your pedal revolutions. Known as revolutions per minute (rpm), cadence is a key component of efficient cycling. Tons of research is out there on cycling cadence and how to use it best for you. For our purposes, we want to pay attention to cadence, establish what a good cadence is for you and where you are riding, and understand what it means.

You can measure cadence in one of two ways: with a bike computer with a cadence meter on your wheel; a power meter (more on this later); or manually counting your rpms. To manually count your cadence, simply hover your right hand over your knee while riding (best done indoors). In ten seconds, count how many times your right knee hits your hand. If it's 8 times, then multiply by 10—that's 80. Your rpm is 80.

An ideal cadence in the cycling world is 90 to 95. I will tell you, that as a beginner, that is *very fast* and something to aspire to. Cadence in the

80s is great for a beginner. While you should work on it (always), don't get bogged down or overly critical of yourself at first. These things take time. Again, this is something to be cognizant of, as it will bear some fruits of improvement as you go along.

Selecting the proper gear for yourself and conditions is paramount to maintaining and working on high cadence. If you have too much/heavy gearing, you will not be capable of spinning fast. This is complicated by outside riding as the terrain changes. For example, if you are on a flat, smooth stretch, then it's easy to pick a gear and focus on cadence. However, once the road starts to pitch up and you are climbing, maintaining that fast cadence must go lockstep with gearing. You still want to "spin up" the hills—as that saves your legs. Just know that this work is a dance, and once you are outside climbing and riding you'll be a-dancin'!

Get Strong!

I did reasonably well as a beginner cyclist because I had strong legs and glutes from all those years of lifting. Despite the extra chub I had put on, I had maintained some muscle power and it helped out big time.

The stronger your legs, the better you will do on the bike—pure and simple. Developing and maintaining a strong core is also important, as the core plays an integral role in riding.

Climbing hills as a heavy rider *is* difficult—simply a matter of physics. You are pulling yourself *up* a hill—bike and all. Lighter riders have less mass to move. Does not mean you can't do it (hell, I finished Lake Placid, Coeur d'Alene, and Louisville Ironmans—all *very* hilly/mountainous courses). But just understand that these types of terrains are tough on heavier riders. Regardless of your size and weight, you must work hard and be strong to do well on hilly courses. Well, flat courses for that matter, too. All courses. Must ride and be strong like bull.

You can build strength in many ways that helps your bike performance: strength training (squats, lunges, thrusters), drills on the bike, riding hill repeats on your bike, and (yes) running. One of my friends and also former coach of mine, Brett Daniels, loves to add "off the bike" squats for his athletes. I loved/hated it so much that I incorporate it into my athlete's workouts, too. It's a little cruel, but does the trick!

Cycling Drills

Like in swimming and running, drills are also a part of a consistent, hard-working cyclist's life. If you are trying to do a triathlon and don't want to get too technical, I totally respect that—and that is also the magic of this book—getting you to your first race without too much number crunching, drama, and details. However, if you want to learn some tools to get faster, be more efficient, cycling drills are the way to go.

Drills *can* be accomplished on an outside ride; however, for the sake of ease and safety, I recommend using a bike trainer or your stationary bike for the execution of drill.

For simplicity's sake, I am including a short list of cycling drills that you can search on Google and explore further if you are ready to kick your cycling up to the next level. These are usually incorporated right after your warm-up, and should be about five to fifteen minutes of your workout. Most drills are like the title sounds: single-leg drill, high-cadence, power intervals, sit-stand intervals, short sprints, 30-second burst drill, and ladder sprints.

Power Meter

A power meter is a large (and probably unnecessary) investment for someone *just starting* in triathlon. However, if you want to take your training to the next level—or you are an advanced cyclist—nothing will do it quicker than riding consistently while having and using your *power* output data to help your training on the bike.

If you aren't someone who will ride consistently, however, don't bother getting a power meter. A power meter won't make you faster—only training will make you faster. If you want to combine training with data—then power meter is the cat's pajamas. Most power meters, depending on the location of the meter, will measure cadence as well, which is why I mentioned it earlier. Power meters can be hub-based (rear wheel), crank-based, bottom-bracket, or pedal-based (dual or single-sided).

A full power meter breakdown isn't for this book; there are some other, great books for the tech savvy who are ready to power up: *Training and Racing with a Power Meter*, by Hunter Allen, Andrew Coggan, and Stephen McGregor (VeloPress, 2018); and *The Power Meter Handbook*, by Joe Friel (VeloPress, 2012).

BASIC BIKE MAINTENANCE
Your LBS (Local Bike Shop)

Establishing a relationship with your local bike shop will make your life so much easier. The cornerstone for a successful relationship with your bike, your LBS will be a great place to learn about your bike, get regular tune-ups, and also just gossip. In the world of triathlon, your LBS is akin to a western saloon—if yours isn't, look for another one, as there is a wild world out there that you are missing. Kidding . . . not really.

You need to have your bike checked out like regular doctor's visits. Cables can stretch, things can creak, and you need to make sure everything is in order. A good time for a first checkup is four to six months after you get your new or new-to-you bike. As you ride, you'll be doing the proper care and love for your bike (riiiiight?), so then once a year or before a big race is a good time for a checkup.

Bike Maintenance Tools and Gear

You can store some tools and such (snacks!) on your bike in bike bags: amazing little bags that fit under your saddle or on your top tube.

In the rear bag, I like to keep the things that do not need to be accessed until I am *off* the bike—think: roadside maintenance. Inside the rear bag: multitool, tire tube(s), tire lever(s), CO_2 cartridge(s) and a CO_2 dispenser—all tools that will help with on-the-road maintenance, including a tube change. Additionally, store some cash in your bag. I like to keep a ten-dollar and also a few one-dollar bills. You never know when you might need some money, and also a dollar bill can be used to assist in changing a flat (Google it!).

Your LBS will be superhandy in letting you know what size tubes and tools you need, how to pump your tires, and more.

Once you have this information, commit it to memory—you will need it.

Keep It Clean

I had a friend who once told me, "You can tell a lot about a person from looking at their underwear drawer." Then another friend said the same about a bike. If you have a crusty and dirty bike, it might say you are sort of a crusty person. Or something like that.

You want your bike in good shape, just like your car. Be good to your bike and she will be good to you.

For starters, it's good practice to clean your bike after any ride outside.

You'll want degreaser, a chain brush, a bucket, and lubricant specific for your bike. Colder-weather riding will require a wax-based lube, whereas summer rides will fare fine with an oil-based lubricant.

For the actual cleaning, you have options: lean it against the side of your house or a brick wall, purchase a standing bike racks (the kind you see at your LBS), or simply put your bike on your car rack to clean it—does the trick! You will need access to a garden hose, preferably with one of those amazing spray nozzles with all the settings. Get a bucket of soap and water. Dish soap works fine—just be mindful of what you are using outside for your yard and the environment—I like the "green" soaps for bike use. Scrub her down with a rag or luxurious bath sponge fit for the princess that is your bike and wash her off.

With the bike washing, you are trying to make her pretty, sure. However, grime and dirt and such is the enemy of a smooth and fast ride. After you wash the bike, check out your chain and see how it's faring. If the chain is really gritty and greasy, it might be time to break out the degreaser. Carefully spray on the degreaser and let it settle for a few minutes. You can then use an old rag or brush to remove the grease.

Once your chain is clean, it's important to re-lube it with proper chain lube. The old faithful White Lightning is a great and inexpensive lube. For application, simply drip-drop lube on the chain as you rotate the pedal around and shift gears. (This is why it's good to have the bike *off* the ground. Otherwise, just pick up the rear wheel with one hand and turn the pedals with the other.) The rotation will share the shiny, new lube around the gears and the chain. Don't forget to wipe off the excess. Like most things in life, moderation plays a fundamental role. If you overlube, you'll get a thick gunky mess that is no fun for later cleanup.

MANICURE PUBLIC SERVICE ANNOUNCEMENT

Ladies, you may love your long, fancy manicured fingernails, but riding a bike with long nails may not love you. At a minimum, get rid of the acrylic, gel, or whatever long nails are of the day. If you ever need to change a tire tube or do other bike maintenance, you just might snap off your talons at the elbows.

Most important, the money you don't spend on the manicure, you can spend on shiny new bike things. See? Brilliant.

In Which I Change a Tube for the First Time

Here's some fun news: when you get a flat tire, the bike "tire" is not the thing that goes flat. Turns out that a bike wheel is like an onion—with several layers.

Your bike tire most likely consists of a rubber tube *inside* the outer rubber tire. The tire holds the tube onto the rim. The tube is what you fill with air—not the tire.

The rim is the shiny metal part of your wheel. The wheel is what fits onto the bike frame. The spokes are what goes into the wheel.

I am not being condescending. I am being serious. I had no idea that to repair your tire tube, you had to take the tire tube *out* of the actual tire. (Something ridiculously difficult to do, by the way.)

A "flat" is actually the tube inside of the tire being punctured, pinched, or a victim of explosion. (I do not kid).

I hate to stereotype, but years of experience requires the next sentence: the vast majority of us are *idiots* at bike maintenance. No matter how many pink books people write about bike maintenance for women, for some reason most of us glaze over when we hear about maintenance. You are not alone if you fall into this camp. For years, I had no real idea how my bike worked. But then I did, because I cared about it, and it's important to learn.

About five months into riding, I figured that I should probably refresh my tube-changing skills. Suffice it to say that forty-five minutes later, I was covered in grease, the curse words were flying, and I was almost in tears—and no tube had been changed. The back-derailleur situation was absolutely befuddling. My CO_2 dispenser was apparently for a mountain bike or a four-wheeler or a horse (nice work, out-of-town bike shop, recommending that *expensive* contraption to the dumb baby lady triathlete).

I was thankful that the Expert did not mock me too badly when I tackled my tube-changing independence. I appreciated him shouting things like, "No, not like that" and nicely telling me to calm down and be a big girl (thanks), and that I needed to know how to maintain my bike. I also appreciated his pretty much telling me exactly *how* to change my tube.

After way too much ado, the tube was changed and I was feeling rightfully proud.

I said, "Ta-da!" showing him my bike.

"Ta-da, what?" the Expert said.

"I did it. The tube is changed. I did it!" I squealed.

The Expert smiled, "Well, you don't know if you've changed it *correctly* until you ride it."

"What?" I asked.

(Truth.)

HOW TO CHANGE A TUBE

The best way to learn to change a tube is by watching online videos or attending an LBS training. Changing a tube is truly easier to watch than read, so we will spare the words.

COMMON CYCLING ISSUES AND HOW TO AVOID THEM
God Save the Queen

I have been through this in nauseating detail. But for a refresher: get the Queen a good saddle, make sure your fit is proper, lube her up, and get a nice, chamois-padded short to wear.

For all of the above, she'll thank you later.

Road Rash

Road rash is slang for the scrapes and abrasions resulting from your sweet lady skin hitting the hard, evil pavement. How to avoid it? Don't fall. But if you do fall, get up quickly, smile, and point at your riding partner. Take proper care of the wounds and get seen by the doc if it's more than a few boo-boos.

Hand and Foot Numbness

Numbness in the hand resulting from cycling occurs often in the small and ring fingers. This numbness may be caused by too much or too long of a pressure on the handlebars. Keep your upper body as relaxed as possible during a ride. Do not ride with your hands gripping the handle-bars like death, with your elbows locked and shoulders to your ears, or with your jaw clenched tight. Relaxation nation, dude. Ride free. That might help the numbness factor.

Foot and toe numbness may also become an issue. This may be caused by improper bike fit and equipment. Sometimes being too far back/forward/up/down in the saddle puts pressure on your nerves and causes numbness in the feet.

Another possible issue causing the numbness might be the position of the cleats (the snap-in clip on the bottom of the bike shoe). Moving the cleat as far back on the shoes as possible (toward the heel) may help. Your shoes may be too big, too small, or the toe straps too tight.[3] A harder soled bike shoe might also help alleviate numbness.

Any sort of numbness or strangeness in the body while riding, in my experience, is usually tied to bike fit or faulty equipment. Rarely is it a medical condition that requires a lot of worry—but of course, be cautious. If you are concerned with the numbness or other issues, certainly see your health-care practitioner, say you are a cyclist, and get a checkup. Regard-less, stay the course and continue troubleshooting these issues. You'll find a solution—sometimes it just takes longer than you'd like.

Lower-Back, Hip, and Knee Discomfort

Many lower-back and knee pains from cycling go back to bike fit and shoe fit. If you have had your bike fitted by a professional *several times* and are still uncomfortable or having back and knee pains, then you should go to *another* professional.

A bike seat that is too low can result in knee pain on the front of the knee, especially if you are riding a lot of hills. A bike seat that is too high can cause knee and hip pains in different locations, as well as lower back strain. Keep working on the bike fit. And if that fails, then go to your doctor. Then, back to another bike professional.

Remember to relax. And do not ride like a circus unicyclist—keep those knees in to help prevent potential knee pain.

Cramping on the Bike

Remember to stay hydrated while you are riding. Cycling is the longest discipline out of the three and you may be out in the heat and sunlight for hours. Get extra water bottle cages, fill your bottles often, use hydration/electrolyte tablets, and drink. Lack of hydration can lead to cramping and worse—so, stay hydrated and properly electrolyted.

8 THE RUN

RUNNING HAS ALWAYS BEEN WEIRD FOR ME. I WAS AN ADULT-onset runner, not running much as a child. I tend to flail. My legs do not leave the ground quickly or smoothly or easily. Even now, after achieving some pretty big goals, I do not run like the wind. I do not run like a breeze, even. But I *do* run, and that is something—actually, it is *everything*. Because all you need to do to become a runner? Well, just run.

If you are starting out or if you feel like absolute crap about yourself, you can choose today to change. Even if you want to cry every single morning because of the shape you are in, you *must* start *somewhere*. And lucky for you—today is the day to run!

Eventually, if you are consistent, you will be one of those crazy people who love to run. I can call you crazy because I am one of you. *I'm Meredith and I am no natural-born runner and I love to run. (For a refresher on this, see pages 44–45, a.k.a. "that time I started running and got bruises on the bottom of my feet.")*

Consistency? It's a big thing, and eventually things get easier and even the unlikeliest of runners *can* become runners.

I changed. Me—the gal who liked to wear sweaters in the summer to hide her body. The lesson? People *can* change. And people can change for the *better*. And with triathlon, you will change. Learn to love who you are becoming. By making small steps, you *are* changing. Learn to appreciate the journey because it is *your* journey.

Every day will get better. Each day *you* will get better, inside and out. Your runs will get longer and stronger. And you will be a runner. That's good stuff.

I asked Gerry to contribute to the Run section of this book, because truly he is one of the great inspirations in my triathlon life. Also, he's a fast runner. Street cred—it's a thing.

Gerry began his triathlon journey in his mid-thirties, looking for a way to extend his ability to compete and stay fit. Gerry worked hard to achieve some impressive goals: qualifying for and competing in the IRONMAN World Championship for both the full and 70.3 distance. Along the way, he became a coach and has helped athletes of all ages, backgrounds, and ability levels achieve their triathlon goals. The dude is the real deal—even though he remains ridiculously humble about it all.

Gerry has coached me off and on for the vast majority of my triathlon "career," and the reason for that is he understands a fundamental belief of mine: *there is more to life than triathlon.* You see, as you get better and faster in the sport, sometimes it's easy to lose perspective on *life*—you can forget how much training is important, but that it is not everything. Gerry has always helped me maintain good perspective, and for that, I am grateful.

Here, Gerry has agreed to share his wisdom on the third (and most wicked) discipline of triathlon: the run.

GO SLOW TO GO FAST

by Gerry Halphen

Remember two very important things when you begin a running program, especially in triathlon:

Go Slow to Go Fast
and
Focus on *Quality* Instead of Quantity

What does "go slow to go fast" really mean? It means to take your time, build a solid foundation of good running form, and develop the proper running habits. It also means to run slow—to later go faster, as we'll discuss.

As a beginner, you should not attempt to go from the couch to a marathon in a week. That's like the binge diet of triathlon training—it won't work, and you'll be sorry later. You may run 26 miles, but you'll certainly end up in the ER.

Going slow *does* work. If you structure your training in a methodical way, the simple adaptations to your body will happen to make you a better runner. Eventually, the speed will follow. This methodology takes time and patience to build and varies by individual. Many different things—such as bodyweight and stressors in life—may impact your progress. But this method is proven: if you have enough time and go slowly, your body will adapt over time and what appears to be impossible—will become real.

The next important component is to maintain *quality* workouts. If you can give fifteen minutes of high quality, then I will take that any day over an hour of crappy effort. If you focus on the *quality* of your time in your running shoes, eventually, the *quantity* will take care of itself.

The Gear

You've read Meredith on this, and I'm going to say it again: go to a running store that will take time to do a shoe fit. Experts at excellent running stores will watch you run on treadmill or run outside the store before attempting to put you in a shoe. They will use their analysis of your gait, foot strike, and other factors to put you in the right shoe which makes all the difference.

Different theories exist about how often you should replace your shoes. I have found that having a rotation of running shoes is nice. Once you find a pair you like, then purchase a few pairs and rotate them. Typically, the rule is to replace shoes every 500 miles, but this will vary wildly depending on foot strike, shoe, and weight of the athlete.

Your choice of sock is really all about feel. Some athletes like ultrathin socks; some like more padding. You will know after trying a few pairs. Regardless, you will want to pick up a specialty running sock, not just a typical cotton tube sock. Whether you like thick or thin socks, a running sock will be made of more breathable material that will help to prevent chafing and blisters in the long run.

Running Surfaces

For a new runner or triathlete, running on a mixture of surfaces is a great idea for variety, strength, and overall running health. This includes running on a trail, other soft surface, treadmill, *and* pavement. You're better off starting with a majority of your runs on soft surfaces, but you must mix in the pavement because most races take place on pavement. This does not mean that you need to zoom on the pavement. You still need to go slow to go fast. If you spend too much time on the pavement to start, you can injure yourself from the pounding. Be smart about where you run and listen to your body. Still, remember to work in the pavement running, because if you run on nothing but soft surface, then your legs will break down on pavement in a race.

I know some people who do all their training on treadmills. Speaking as a coach, minute for minute a treadmill creates a precision with training that you simply cannot obtain from outside running, where such distractions as cars, stop lights, and so on can disrupt a run. Further, if you are pressed for time as most women are, the treadmill is the perfect solution. You get up to speed quickly, are forced to hold the pace (hello: the belt is moving!), and you can vary your "terrain" as needed with the incline settings.

You'll hear people call it the "dreadmill." They'll whine, "I can't run on the dreadmill for more than twenty minutes!" The longest run I have done on a treadmill is 22 miles. Was it mentally draining? Of course, it was. Running on a treadmill can make you want to poke out your eyes. Which is precisely the point of doing it! To build *mental endurance*.

Running Form

As with shoes, there are many theories about running form. Especially for a beginner, I firmly believe that it is more important to go out and be active and get some miles in your legs than to have the perfect form. If you are waiting on the perfect form, then you will come up with the excuse "I can't run because my form's not good."

At the same time, you need to balance the mileage with the *quality* of your workout. There it is again. *quality*. Good running form makes you a more efficient runner. Being efficient saves energy and allows your mind to be present, working, and sharp when you need it.

If you get very fatigued from the beginning, your central nervous system begins to wane, and you can make bad decisions, both in training and on race day.

Some helpful things to remember that will improve your running technique:

1. **Work on your core and lower back strength.** Maintaining a strong back and core has everything to do with maintaining posture and proper form. The back and the core are often components that people neglect, but they are quite literally the center of power. By your engaging your core, your legs will not suffer (as much). Therefore, when it comes time to run, you have better running form.

2. **Keep your feet underneath your body.** Your stride should be reasonably short, meaning to keep your feet under your body. An extended (too long) stride will add stress on your back, knees, and hips. If your feet remain *under* your body, then you will turn over your feet more quickly and propel yourself forward faster.

3. **Foot strike.** There are many different arguments on heel strike versus foot strike. Again, it is important for a new runner to hit the road and begin moving. Still, working on keeping your feet beneath you during the run will help prevent a hard-to-break heel strike habit later. The heel strike, if it is deliberate enough, will serve to actually slow you down and "brake" your run stride.

4. **Relax your body.** As when you're on the bike, you want to relax your upper body, right down to your jaw. This includes your hands.

5. **Posture.** Have excellent posture, but you want to lean your body ever so slightly forward *from the ankles*. In other words, picture a straight line from your ankles through your body. That line should stay straight and rotate slightly forward during your run.

6. **Get rid of the chicken wing.** Keep your arms close to your body and don't flail them around like a chicken. (Ah-hem, Meredith.)

7. **Consider giving Galloway a try.** The Galloway Method[1] of running has proven some great results for beginners and advanced athletes alike. Basically, Galloway is about incorporating walking breaks into your running sessions (and races). You can run for five minutes, then walk for one minute; run for a mile, walk for a minute—whichever combination you choose is up to you. It's important to note that Jeff Galloway provides a "formula" for his time-tested, most effective run-walk intervals on his website, JeffGalloway.com. The secret to the method (like most things) is consistency. No matter what intervals you use and train with, then simply stick to that plan and implement it. If the formula doesn't work for your body, you can try changing up the intervals until you have found your consistent intervals. If, after much trying, you just are not sticking with any of the run-walk intervals you set out to use, then maybe it's not for you. The Galloway Method is just that—a method—and methodology only works when it's followed.

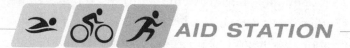

AID STATION

Meredith here. During my third Ironman race in Louisville, I set out to run the marathon with a three-minute run followed by a one-minute walk. This was simply *the* most consistent long-distance run of my life. I managed to hold a great pace, feel well, and go on to finish the marathon in just over six hours—which is a great time for an IRONMAN marathon for me.

If you feel that running "isn't for you," seriously give Galloway run-walk a try—it is a game-changer for the adult-onset runners.

Add Drills

To improve your form, basic running drills may be incorporated into your training. The Internet has an endless catalog of videos for various running drills. You can see the demonstrations for drills, such as 100 ups (Chris McDougall featured by the *New York Times* online[2]), carioca, A skips, B skips, high-knees, straight-leg bounds, quick feet, jump hop hop, dynamic monster walks, lateral squats, and more. All of the foregoing are fun ways to improve the running motion.

Build Your Endurance

One of the most common misconceptions is that you have to go hard all the time to improve. The more I do triathlon, the more I have come to understand just how important low-intensity training is. As I mentioned before, you want to *go slow* in order to *go fast* later.

This method of training is based on heart rate zones. You monitor your zones through the use of a heart rate monitor (usually worn on the wrist) and a chest strap (which fastens around your chest, just under the bottom of your sports bra band). The chest strap reads the heart rate and transmits the data to the watch. New technology has heart rate capabilities built into the watch or device itself, or there are other options to wear on the wrist and more coming. While there are several methodologies for structuring the actual heart rate training, ranging from four to seven target zones, I've included the simpler four-zone method here for illustration purposes.

Maintaining your runs in Zone 2 or approximately 70 to 80 percent of your maximum heart rate (or 80% to 90% of your lactate threshold) will build endurance. Lactate threshold is determined by blood lactate testing (BLT) and is the most accurate way to determine your specific heart rate zones.

If all else fails, you can *broadly* estimate your heart rate zones (though this is a very generalized method and most experts would agree not to rely on this) by using 220 minus your age for your maximum heart rate. Although most fitness practitioners agree that this method is crude and can be off by 10 percent or more, if you are just getting into exercise, it is a place to start. As you get more into the discipline of training and if you want more precision with your heart rate zones, I'd recommend conducting a BLT.

To improve endurance, you must build both your aerobic base *and* your anaerobic (muscular) endurance. You improve your *aerobic* endur-

HEART RATE ZONES

Zone 1—active recovery, beginner programs (60% to 70% of your max heart rate)

Zone 2—endurance and aerobic base building (70% to 80% of your max heart rate)

Zone 3—aerobic and anaerobic combination (often I refer to Zone 3 as no-man's-land, because you are not completely aerobic, nor are you anaerobic; 80% to 90% of your max heart rate)

Zone 4—anaerobic threshold (where a beginner does not want to be; 90% to 95% of your max heart rate)

Again, there are several methodologies that go up to seven different zones, but we are using Zone 4 for the sake of simplicity for a beginner. Additionally, the BLT is the best way to determine your proper zones! However, if you *must* use the broad estimator, here is an example using a 33-year-old woman: 220 minus 33 equals an *estimated* maximum heart rate = 187 beats per minute.

Based on 187 as a maximum heart rate, her zones were calculated as follows:

Zone 1: 112–130 (60% to 70%)

Zone 2: 131–149 (70% to 80%)

Zone 3: 150–168 (80% to 90%)

Zone 4: 169–177 (90% to 95%)

ance by going slowly, staying in Zone 2, particularly *low* Zone 2, during your runs. This practice will expand not only your aerobic capacity, but it will allow time for your body to adapt to the training, the movements and the shock you might be putting it through. By the way, as a bonus, this time in low Zone 2 will also maximize your fat burning as your body can/will use fat as a fuel source at this lower level of exertion.

Conversely, you build your *anaerobic* engine by going hard, sprinting, or doing hill climb repeats, or quick, heavy strength moves. Therefore, by expanding and working both systems—you have two stronger engines.

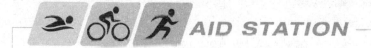 AID STATION

Endurance is the ability to go farther and longer.

When you think about having lots of endurance—think about the ability to run farther than just one mile super-fast—think about running five, six or twenty-six miles and being *able* to do so well. Endurance is built slowly and with time. Eventually endurance *and* speed mesh—creating the ability to go far *and* fast.

Both of these magic things, however, take time. So be patient!

It is rare to find an athlete, especially one who thinks she's fast, who can agree to turn down the "heat" and run slow according to a low Zone 2. But this type of training pays huge dividends.

There is another method of training intensity monitoring called rate of perceived exertion (RPE). This method is based on how you feel. The correlation is typically as follows:

Heart Rate Zone	RPE
Zone 1	easy
Zone 2	moderate
Zone 3	slightly difficult
Zone 4	extremely difficult

This may be a good way to train as a beginner, but I recommend using the heart rate method as soon as possible on your journey, as it will yield more accurate results. That being said, you should always be in tune with your "perceived exertion"—no matter what you are doing—and adjust accordingly.

As a new triathlete, you will want to spend plenty of time going slow. You might think: *That's the only speed I've got!* Well, even better, then! Even later as you get stronger and faster, you will want to continue to incorporate slow runs into your training. Slow runs continue to improve your aerobic base as well as allow you to focus on a smooth, clean running form. You will want to also incorporate short, fast runs and hill workouts, which will increase your muscular strength, improve your foot speed, and build your anaerobic engine. It's training *both* the aerobic and anaerobic engines that yield the best long-term results.

Warm Up to Run

I do not believe in static stretching before a run. I prefer walking or jumping jacks, or other forms of "dynamic stretching."

Examples of dynamic stretches are side lunge, leg swings, single-leg deadlifts, glute activators, butt kicks, skips, and high knees. You can also use these to warm up for cycling as well.

Side lunge: With your feet facing forward and shoulder width apart, take a deep, wide step to your right. Bend your left knee as you shift your weight over your right foot. Return to the middle and standing. Repeat for 40 seconds, then switch sides.

Leg swings: With this stretch, you can cover all the leg swings: straight, bent knee forward and lateral. They are just as they sound— with your hand on a wall for stability, you are swinging your legs in a fluid motion for 10 to 12 repetitions, and switching legs. One leg is bearing body weight, and the other is swinging—either straight legged laterally, bent knee laterally (using the hips), or bent knee forward.

Single-leg deadlift: Stand on your left leg with your knee slightly bent. Slowly hinge forward until your torso and right leg are parallel to the floor. Return to standing. Repeat for 30 seconds, then switch sides.[3]

Glute activators: One of the things I learned from sitting at a desk for years was that my butt had essentially stopped working. Apparently, we use our butts a lot in running (*if* we are doing it correctly). Practice squeezing your glutes and also alternating the squeeze from cheek to cheek to activate those muscles. If nothing works when you try this, you might have the dreaded "dead butt"—which means these activation exercises are even more important. Time to wake your butt up!

Butt kicks, skips, and high-knees: You have probably seen these drills in your own life or on the high school football field. But they are just as they sound and can be a great warm-up. For butt kicks, you want to move forward while kicking your legs behind you with your heels trying to kick your own butt. The skips are a form of movement that looks like childhood skipping, except you are raising that knee in the air higher to simulate a big run push-off. Next, high knees is also a forward motion, but you are pulling your knees high, one at a time, as you move forward. An easy internet search reveals videos of these.

Staying Injury-Free

The easiest way to stay healthy and injury-free is to limit the frequency of running (or swimming or biking, too!), particularly the frequency of *intense* running (or swimming or biking). You do *not* need to run as much as people think. For example, since I started this sport fifteen years ago, I have managed (during my training times) to get faster every year by running no more than three times a week. And that includes my IRONMAN training. What you do in those runs will vary depending on what distance race you are attempting, but the key point—wait for it—is that *quality* matters more than *quantity*.

Additionally, most bodies have difficulty tolerating running more than three times a week—the body may break down and open itself up for injury. Regardless, no matter how much or how little you are running, you need to listen to your body. If you are hurting or exhausted, then you may need some recovery time.

Remember to work on your strength training and core. I have provided some diverse types of exercises. The type and duration of strength and core should change throughout the season, but it should always be a mainstay of your training.

I also recommend an ice bath after any effort beyond an hour. Yes, I said ice bath. While horrific and medieval, ice baths are essential.

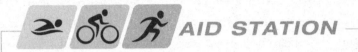

AID STATION

Overuse injuries are very common in beginner runners. From shin splints to pulled muscles to actual stress fractures in the foot and legs, taking the advice to run no more than three times a week is sound for the new runner. You can always amp up the intensity and volume later—don't get hurt and derail your goals from overuse. A little common sense goes a long way.

While this is purely anecdotal, though I am sure there is some research to support it, having excellent nutrition and sleep quality is a big factor in staying injury-free for the long haul as well.

Finally, find the new love of your life: the foam roller. There are many types of rollers and tools on the market now. Using the foam roller is a form of self-massage and myofascial release that works like a deep tissue massage. This practice hurts, but is a fantastic training longevity tool.

If you do not know what an IT band is now, you will when you start running. The term stands for "iliotibial band," which is a "band" of tissue that runs along the outside of the thigh, over the hip, down the knee, and below the knee. Essentially, the IT band's job is keep the knee stable during walking and running.

One of the best ways to *help* the IT band when it starts to act up is to exert pain *on* the IT band, by rolling on a foam roller (in all directions), using a stick roller (also, all directions), a lacrosse ball or trigger-point ball, getting a deep tissue massage; embarking on active release technique therapy (ART[4]), or doing whatever you can to work that IT band loose. Remember to roll up and down as well as horizontally—to work the whole band. Please note that, in recent times, the IT band has gotten a bad rap and tends to be over abused with therapy. Definitely take the time to get evaluated by a specialist before you go too hard on your IT band.

Run Workouts

I recommend a simple breakdown for the three weekly run workouts:

"Long" Run
Moderate Run
Hard Run

The "Long" Run

This is your aerobic building run/jog/walk, which consists of going long and slow, in a low Zone 2 heart rate zone. Long runs, known as "base-building" runs, create the foundation of your aerobic system. Of course, starting out the "long" run may not feel very long but the idea is to have a long(er) run each week.

Remember: you go slow and long in order to go fast. On the long run workouts, you should focus on your heart rate and your running technique. If you cannot run *and* keep your heart rate in Zone 2, then you should walk (as fast as you can) and focus on your heart rate staying in Zone 2. You will build up to a jog eventually—and yes, then a run. (See more about the Galloway Method on page 138.)

The benefit of this Long Run workout is to build your aerobic base. This base will be built by keeping your heart rate under control—again, even if this means walking. You want to keep the mileage *high* and the heart rate *low*. Focus on the quality of each stride.

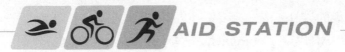

AID STATION

A FIRST LONG RUN

Meredith here. My first 8-mile run showed up on the training schedule and I was perplexed. Eight miles was a really, really long way.

The good thing about the park and the loop course I chose was the bathroom. I do not mean that anything special was happening with this bathroom, but rather the good thing was the mere *presence* of the bathroom.

On Mile 4.5, I thought I would be forced to dodge into the bushes. The stomach cramping. The rumblings. *Oh no oh no oh no.* I stumbled the half mile back around to the bathroom at the park. I was prairie-dogging, puckering, and limping—all the moves I could muster to hold it all in. As I crashed into the bathroom, I thought, *I guess I'm done with this run.*

Then I thought, *Well, if I was in a race, I'd have to keep going or get picked up by the quit-mobile.*

I started some serious self-talk babble. Self-talk babble always begins with the word *well*.

Well, I can surely run 2.5 miles and finish this up! Yes, I can!

This self-talk was happening while I was hovering over the toilet and playing peek-a-boo with a toddler who was sticking his head under the stall door.

Yes, you can. Yes, you can.

Then I thought, *Well, what if I pass out? What if I fall down? What if I actually poop my pants this time?*

But really, there was no time for negative talk. I needed to get home. I needed to make my ten o'clock conference call. I needed to get a move on, one way or the other. After three or so more minutes in the john, the toddler was gone, the cramping had slowed, and I felt semi-normal.

I grinded out the final 2.5, limping the last bit and brought it home. *Eight miles.*

I could not believe it. I did it! Hours later I was so thankful that I did not walk off the loop that day. I gave it everything I had. Even though, I really, really wantod to hang that one up. Even though my body had given up on me. Even though I almost pooped my pants.

The Moderate Run

On this particular workout day, you should incorporate some increases in pace (intervals) and also, where possible, running on hills. The purpose of the moderate run is to use both your aerobic *and* anaerobic engines.

For example: complete a thirty-minute workout, while every five minutes picking up the pace or going uphill for one or two minutes, holding steady, then dropping down for a few minutes of recovery. Repeat until the thirty minutes is up. As you get more advanced, you can add longer intervals, steeper hills and/or less recovery.

The Hard Run

Hard run is a relative term depending on your experience level. If you are a brand-new runner (or even walker), *intensity* means one thing. If you are a young, seasoned 800-meter runner on a sports scholarship, it means something else. It is important to have a clear idea of your intensity levels and to remember that yes, it will be hard. But a "hard run" is hard regardless of whether you are a newbie or the experienced athlete. Hardness depends on your *personal* level, but can be measured fairly easily by the rate of perceived exertion scale or heart rate. For RPE, the "hard" intervals or runs (depending on how the workout is written) can be characterized as an 8, 9, or 10 on the scale. Your heart rate zones will likely be high, Zone 3 and into 5, during some points of the workout. Read: the puke level should be high.

An example of a hard run workout could be a 5K test run. Warm up for ten minutes, then run 3.1 miles as hard and as fast as you can do it. This is often used as a heart rate test by coaches (called field testing). Another hard workout could incorporate track work, longer and harder intervals than your moderate run, or high-intensity hill repeats. Here you may do some of the same types of workouts as the moderate run, but at a higher intensity.

As a true beginner runner, however, it's best to stick to only slower runs for a few months. Why? Well, for starters, any running will feel "hard" enough. Again, you want to stay injury-free as well. Just keep moving along at the slower pace and eventually, you will be able to differentiate between the three types of runs.

If you build your aerobic base and then omit the moderate and hard runs, your anaerobic (muscular) base will decrease (as well as your running potential). While these two types of runs add variety to the training and make it more interesting, they also serve to confuse your body and prevent the ever-dreaded plateau.

With regard to completing a run as long as the "race distance" *before* your race, this absolutely depends on the athlete. For example, do you mentally feel the need to run a 5K before you do a sprint triathlon? I believe you can benefit from having run 4 or 5 miles before a sprint triathlon, but it is not essential. Most athletes benefit from knowing in the back of their mind that they can do the same distance of the run in the race *before* race day. At the same time, you can certainly run a 5K in a triathlon if you have run 3.1 miles in training.

Remember that the sum of the parts is greater. If you maximize the quality of all three events (swim, bike, and run), you will be rested and can feed off the adrenaline of the race. One of the key sayings in triathlon is: the hardest part is getting to the *starting line*. That also means getting to the starting line intact, without injury.

The Brick Workout

As Meredith explained earlier, running immediately after you bike is known as a brick. This is an important component of your training because the brick workout simulates the physical and mental stressors on your race day. You must train your legs to get accustomed to the feeling of coming off the bike and immediately running. Trust me—it never feels "normal"—but the more you do it, the more easily your body agrees to adapt.

After you have built a solid aerobic foundation, I recommend making one of your run workouts a week a brick; where you run anywhere from 1 to 4 miles *after* your bike workout. This varies from race distance to race distance, but a sprint and Olympic distance would be served well with this rule of thumb. The distance is not as important as the body adaptation to the feeling of "bricks" in your legs as you run off the bike.

Saving Yourself for the Run in the Race

The energy for the last part of a triathlon is greatly about mental preparation and mental control. Sure, you need physical endurance, but you must control your output during the first two segments (the swim and the bike) with the knowledge you still must complete the last segment of the race: the run.

In training, utilizing the brick workouts will help your body learn to adapt to the cumulative fatigue of running when you are tired. The brick workouts are a superb foundation for being able to tolerate and adapt to the run at the end of the race. Using your mind to control your body starts in training, and adapting to the fatigue is another part of this.

9 OTHER IMPORTANT TRAINING STUFF

STRETCHING

For your preworkout stretching, try something to get the blood flowing—such as jumping jacks, burpees, or dynamic stretching. You may need to put on your diaper for any jumping after childbirth—just saying. Dynamic stretching (e.g., the running drills outlined in the prior chapter) is helpful, especially in the shoulders. You essentially utilize a full range of movement, such as a swim stroke or shoulder circles, and repeat to warm up.

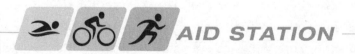

AID STATION

If you do, in fact, tinkle a little when you jump, often this is simply indicative of pelvic floor weakness—from age, or childbirth. You can strengthen your transverse abdominals, your core (see page 152), and your pelvic floor with some easy exercises (check Google!) or see a pelvic floor specialist. It can get better with just a little work.

Stretching *after* a workout and on recovery days is vitally important. This is where static stretching comes in: the slow, methodical method of stretching (no bouncing). You pick a muscle group—hamstrings, for instance—and attempt to touch your toes, moving as gradually as you can to achieve the best (but not painful) stretch possible. Static stretching is best saved for *after* a workout or on recovery days. I like a combination of standard hamstring, hip flexor, and quad static stretches for my lower body with the use of lacrosse balls, rollers, and sticks. Then, I use the foam roller to "roll out" my IT band (see page 144), hamstrings, and calves. I use shoulder rolls, triceps stretches, and other shoulder stretches for my upper body.

A big part of triathlon training includes proper stretching, fascia release, and massage techniques. You will find that stretching is a matter of personal preference, but you must find what works for you. Find it, and use it. Stretching and foam rolling are vital to your triathlon habit.

STRENGTH AND STABILITY
Core

The midsection, abs, and back muscles are often referred to as your core—these are the muscles that support your spine and keep your body stable and balanced. You might be surprised to learn that your core stretches all the way to your lady parts—the mystery that is the "pelvic floor" is part of your core.

A tough midsection and lower back is necessary for smoothness in the water, holding form on the bike, and your posture during the run. Apparently, a strong core is the secret to solving all the world's problems, in addition to being the foundation of the body and all of its movements.

So, basically, because the core is so important, I was introduced to the hideousness that is known as . . . the *plank*.

While there are a million different resources available out there for core moves, core strength and the like, the most powerful of all is the plank. I really can't even talk about a plank without feeling shame and fear. It is so hard!

It looks like a push-up on your forearms, except you are not moving. I'm sure you've seen it. If not, ask Google. You'll see, and once you *do*, you'll *feel*.

A plank is performed as follows:

- Lie on the floor, facedown, with your forearms on the floor.
- Push up off the floor as if doing a push-up, but instead of completing a push-up, rest on your forearms and elbows.
- Keeping your back as flat as possible, engage your core muscles to prevent your stomach or hips from sagging, or your butt from sticking up in the air.

If you feel it in your back, stop. Take smaller and shorter efforts. There are derivations of the plank: plank with knee raises, side plank, plank with rotation. All are core-busting.

In addition to planks, you should incorporate abdominal moves, such as crunches, leg raises, crunches on a giant ball, sit-ups, V-ups, crunches with weights overhead; stability exercises, such as kettlebell swings; and weightlifting —as long as you are mindful about said core engagement.

Strength and Stability

You can pick up any issue of a fitness magazine and find perfectly acceptable strength workouts—for looking *hot*. But interestingly enough, strength training for triathlon is *different* (and it should be). I don't want to bore you with weight-training and strengthening exercises in this book, but only for one reason: I loathe picking up a book about triathlon and finding half the book to be strength workouts.

I'm like, "Where's the value?! I want to know about *running*, not lunges! I know about lunges! Errrr! *Fitness* has covered lunges for the last twelve issues!"

So, as a beginner, if I picked up a triathlon-centered book, I wanted someone to tell me about swimming, biking, and running—and that's all. But I will admit when I am wrong—and my attitude about strength training in triathlon has been *wrong*. In fact, there is yet another discipline to triathlon: strength training. And I had to learn this the hard way.

In the beginning of my triathlon journey, I was plagued with weird injuries and strange *imbalances* in my body. If right knee hurt, then my left hip started killing me. My back, then my quads. These bizarre issues did not seem to arise until I hit some major mileage in my tri training.

At first I sort of glossed over the importance of strength training. But then, my injuries got worse. At last, an epiphany slapped me in the face: my imbalance issues and injuries could have been prevented *from the start* of my triathlon training.

And interestingly, while swimming, biking, and running did, indeed, make me a triathlete, I needed the balance and foundation brought from strength training to *continue* my triathlon journey. I would not be a triathlete for long, continuing as I was. I was all out of balance.

A triathlon friend turned me on to the book *Holistic Strength Training for Triathlon*, by Andrew Johnston—*the* strength training book specifically for triathlon. I cannot even begin to reference and cite some of the wealth of information that he provides. The book covers the *why* of strength training (and it's not all with weights!), takes you through the *how*, and then some. Take some time to pick up his book and work toward building the strong foundation you need from the beginning of your training.

One of the good things about triathlon strength training (as shown in Johnston's book) is that you can incorporate strength moves for each discipline that do *not* necessarily require hitting the weight room.

Many basic strength moves are floor or standing moves with bodyweight only: no weights needed; exercises, such as pelvic bridge, hip extensions, flexions, and twists; and a variety of stances. These serve to build strength *and* stability from the ground up—starting with your feet, engaging your core, and building a well-rounded body.

Of course, there are strengthening moves *among* the three disciplines, too. In the pool, you can increase your strength by performing swimming sets using a pull buoy or float. That move helps to stabilize your lower body and cause you to rely more on your upper body. The same can be said for hand paddles, although the jury is still out on whether these are good for beginners. You can use a band around your ankles to engage your core—and help you if you are ever thrown off a pirate ship and need to swim away.

On the bike, all you need is your favorite big gear on a flat road or some "suffering" in the hills on your trainer or virtual training. Finally, you can increase your power in the run by incorporating hill repeats, interval training, and all sorts of variations of speed work.

You'll be surprised, however, just how much work can be (and should be) done outside of your swimsuit, cycling shoes, and running shoes—and on the floor of your living room on a yoga mat.

You can also take your strength training to the gym with group fitness classes that are strength-based, personal training or group training, or even on the fringe of tri training with Olympic lifting or CrossFit. As with any strength program, you want to start slow and make sure you have a truly qualified instructor or coach. Strength training is a quick way to—er, gain strength—but it is also an easy way to injure yourself if you are not careful, do not recover properly, or fail to learn and utilize proper form.

By limiting this section, I am not deemphasizing the importance of strength training. Quite the opposite—I am recognizing strength is *far* more important and in-depth than I can cover in this book. The foundation of strength is paramount to your tri training, so do not gloss over it. Strength training from the ground up provides you with the base and the balance you need to stay as injury-free as humanly possible and to thrive in triathlon.

Yoga

Yoga is awesome for core building, stretching, and overall mind and body connection. I find that time for yoga is tricky because there are so many other workouts to accomplish, but I do *love* the way I feel postyoga. If you have time and want to incorporate yoga—do it.

REST AND RECOVERY

I'm just going to say it: for a working wife and mother and, well, for a woman in general, what in the hell is "rest"? I am *never* rested. *Take a rest.* What? You're speaking another language, stranger!

Still, while sleeping in past 9:30 a.m. has not happened in over eleven years, I can attribute great importance to "recovery" and "rest." Running yourself into the ground, which at times feels like a by-product of being a woman, should not be an attribute of triathlon. Triathlon should *benefit* your life, not complicate it. Of course, at times, triathlon will be a complicating factor. But the goal is to make triathlon a positive stressor—not a sanity killer.

To appreciate your workout days, you must relish your recovery days. To have a reasonably successful race day, you need to train smart. That means giving your muscles, your body, your soul, and your brain a rest from training.

There are typically three types of rest-and-recovery themes.

Rest Day

You can have a day completely *off* from training. A day off is, obviously, a day off. Take advantage of true rest days and really rest. Take care of your extra nontraining errands; spend a family day or whatever else will help recharge your soul for the next day of workouts.

Pssssst! You can also have two days off. Or a week. This is your life. Do what makes you happy, healthy, and sane.

Active Recovery Workouts

Active recovery workouts are low in mileage and intensity. For example, these may be a day where you put out an easy spin on the bike or a slow jog/walk. Active recovery days get your blood flowing, and allow you take some much-needed time to focus on your technique.

Recovery Weeks

When you follow a training plan, usually a recovery week will be included every fourth week or so (depending on the training methodology—some coaches or plans go longer, shorter). The recovery week will dial back your mileage and intensity *for the week*—for you to rest and recover properly before the beating of the next training cycle begins. This usually doesn't mean reduced workouts, just reduced intensity and volume.

NO OVERTRAINING ALLOWED!

On rest days, I tend to be crabby and bloated, because I like the endorphins and sweat expulsion that training days bring. At the same time, triathlon is meant to add to your life, not take away from it—so rest days and recovery weeks are fundamental parts of being a triathlete.

Even when I am crabby, I have learned that I still need the break. On a neuromuscular level, rest days and recovery weeks are vital. It's easier to "survive" the rest days if you look at them as a time to recharge and regroup for your next big workout.

Overtraining is a big danger in triathlon. You can very easily become so focused (obsessed) that you fail to listen to your body, your training plan, or your coach. If you fail to insert recovery into your plan, you are at a risk for physical damage *and* psychological damage (read: complete and utter burnout). Take a break. If you feel overtrained, take another break. Rest until you feel you are ready to go again.

Don't get me wrong: you will be *tired* from training. You may wake up tired. You may go to bed tired. You may fall asleep on the potty. You may sleep at your desk at work (*oh, I mean* . . .). But there is a difference between tired and fatigued. Rest is yet another component of overall health and balance. You need to stay hydrated, mentally focused, happy (as happy as possible), and sane.

Remember *quality* over *quantity* in training. It is far better to take a rest day (even an extra one here and there) to ensure that your next workout is the best workout possible.

A TRAINING PLAN FOR YOUR TRIATHLON

A beginner training plan is a good jumping-off point for you to gain an *idea* of the training, the reasonable time commitment, and to begin to search out your best training plans, coaching, and motivation to get you to your race.

I do implore you to find a coach or a team that can help you—an online plan is no substitute for a person—and the motivation and accountability from *others* is a big part of triathlon. If you cannot hire a coach or do not have access to a club, then I urge you to create your own calendar and do your homework to create your special plan. You can use Google Calendar, or even the free TrainingPeaks.com software. Keep records and hold yourself accountable.

Ultimately, remember that the key is not a magic training plan or a coach, but a determination within yourself, a consistency to complete the workouts, and moving forward the best you can! You will get there.

At the end of this book, Appendix B, I have included a simple training plan for a first triathlon. This section will *not* to give you a foolproof training plan. *Do not tape this training plan to your mirror and hide it in your sports bra and call it gospel.* But *do* look at it, consider the steps, and figure out how to make it work for you. You have two training plan options, depending on where you are in your fitness abilities. They are Plan 1, for a true beginner (off-the-couch) in all three disciplines; and Plan 2, for a fitness geek (someone who is in good shape, but has never completed a triathlon). Depending on where you fall in that spectrum, you can combine the plans. For example, if you are brand new to swimming, but know how to ride and run, then you can incorporate the swim part from Plan 1 into Plan 2 for the bike and run. It will make more sense as you dive into it. Just remember to adjust where it makes sense, have faith, and have fun!

COMING ATTRACTIONS

You would think that the next chapter should be about race day. And I would tend to agree with you.

However, you need to handle more things in your life *before* you get to race day. Important things, such as mental toughness, nutrition, and integrating your training with a job and family. I will cover your race day and preparation, I promise. But first, let's talk about getting your mind, your nutrition, and (if applicable) your family set on your journey.

10 THE MENTAL GAME

MUCH OF TRIATHLON IS TRAINING THE MIND TO TOLERATE the pain that the body is experiencing. But you must not simply *tolerate* pain. Instead, your goal should be to embrace the pain, love it, and make friends with it. Much of triathlon is about embracing and enjoying the pain. I thought this was crazy until I began to practice it . . . and then saw the great results from focusing my mind to endure the hurt. Sometimes even enjoy it.

But triathlon is not *only* about enduring the beating of the training. The training is also about wrapping your head around your true strengths, learning to believe in yourself, and using the sport as a foundation for a better, stronger life. You will learn that you are stronger, faster, and tougher than you ever thought possible if you stay strong of mind and just keep going.

Four vitally important Mental Game Rules must be followed with respect to triathlon.

The Mental Game Rules

Rule #1: Believe in yourself.

Rule #2: Ignore those who do not believe in you.

Rule #3: Know when to stop.

Rule #4: Know when to keep going.

Strength and character can be built from this sport—I know this with all of my heart. Pushing through the pain, the doubt, and the sweat to go to a new place (a run distance, a swim personal record) will reveal more about you . . . *to* you.

You may not believe in yourself right this second, but you must begin thinking in terms of belief. Start out with just once-a-day mind tricks. Once a day, think about triathlon and simply say to yourself, *I can do this.* No need to dwell on it; do it quickly and move on with cooking dinner or driving.

Our mental toughness is born and takes root in our day-to-day thoughts and affirmations. If we are constantly beating ourselves up in our own head, we will believe those thoughts. We must say nice things.

Little by little, add other little affirmations to your day that will help you focus on yourself:

I am a runner.

I like to swim.

Triathlon is changing my life.

I can do this.

I will do this.

I cannot wait for race day.

Triathlon is the bomb, diggity-boogity. Woot woot.

Your mind is the controlling force of your entire body. Use it for your benefit!

PANIC. BIKE. WALK.

This is a tale about overcoming panic.

On the morning of my first-ever open water swim, it was forty-three degrees. The lake was a chilly sixty-two degrees. *Brrrr.*

As we pulled through the gates of the park, I saw Coach Gerry and other people milling about. *Oh no,* I thought. *Others. Real triathletes. And me. And the Expert. No. No no no no.* My heart raced. The Expert parked the car. We fumbled with our gear and wetsuits at the back of the car. The Expert and I had matching wetsuits.

Stupid Orca triathlon sale. Two little love whales.

As I pulled on my suit, the Expert decided to be a Superexpert. Attempting to mimic Gerry's helpful yank on *his* suit, the Expert turned me around and gave my suit a good pull from the rear.

I gasped. "Did you just rip my wetsuit?!" I wailed.

"No. No, uh, no," he mumbled. Pause.

"Yes," he stuttered, "Oh no. I'm sorry!" He was pleading with his puppy dog eyes, looking as shocked as I was.

"Oh, for the love," I mumbled, shooting him dead with open water daggers from my eyes.

I was not mad. Rather, I was absolutely horror-stricken. I had heard of wetsuits being filled with water, followed by sinking and inevitable death. Okay, that's not completely true. But I have heard that a wetsuit can fill up with water. I was freaked.

Panic Number One.

As I walked toward the beach in my holey wetsuit with the Expert and Gerry, I was so freaking nervous. But my subconscious told me that I would be okay. I fastened my swim cap, my goggles. I walked into the lake, up to the ankles. The water was cold. Really cold. *It's okay,* I told myself, *you have been in cold water before.*

I waded up to my thighs, then my belly. I had a flashback to my weightlifting days and the notorious ice baths. The chill took my breath away. The water crept up to my elbows and finally my shoulders. My heart was pounding. *This $^!# is cold. This $^!# is also bananas.*

Then, I put my face in the water. The instant it hit the water, I gasped and inhaled what could only have been the entire lake. I immediately panicked and snapped my head out of the water, sputtering.

Beginner's bad luck. I got this. I stuck my face into the water for a second time. I gasped yet again and inhaled more water into my lungs. My body was fighting me. Each time I placed my face in the water, I tried my best not to inhale, but the reaction was automatic: I sucked in water. *Crap crap crap. $^!#. Bananas. $^!#. Bananas. Crap.*

Gerry gestured out to the lake. "We're going to swim out to that first buoy and then take a left and swim to each of those four buoys and circle back."

I could not breathe.

The pressure on my shoulders and chest from the wetsuit was mind-boggling. I had been warned that the wetsuit would make my chest feel heavy. But I was not prepared for the coffinlike feeling on my chest, my back, my shoulders, and my entire upper body. *Was I having a heart attack? Panic Number Two.*

I am severely claustrophobic. With my face in the dark water, I was certain that I was burying myself alive. *Panic Number Three.* I tried to swim forward, but I could not freestyle. I could not manage to breaststroke, sidestroke, or even float. I was completely paralyzed. I swam three strokes, but then I would shoot up gasping all over again. I saw Gerry 100 meters away, gesturing and shouting, "Just come to the buoy."

If only it were that simple, Iron dude, I thought.

But three strokes at a time, I made it to the buoy. I looked back and saw the Expert. I don't think he was *behind* me, per se. *He* seemed fine. I clawed at the slick sides of the buoy, searching and begging for a place to grab on. *There's nowhere to grab on this damn buoy!* I finally understood why drowning people take down others in the process of their drowning. When I couldn't get a grip on the buoy, it took everything I had inside *not* to wrap my arms around Gerry and use him as a life preserver.

I continued to claw at the buoy, whispering to Gerry, "I. Can. Not. Breathe. I. Need. To. Go. Back." I could not estimate how much water I had swallowed. *Panic Number Four.*

My mind flashed to that scene from *Sex and the City* where Carrie tries on a wedding gown and immediately breaks out into hives and rips the dress off, deciding that she could not possibly get married. I felt exactly that way: *I could not possibly do triathlon.* I needed the freaking wetsuit off my Orca body. I was overwhelmed. *Panic Number Five.*

I could see Gerry's lips moving, but I could not hear him. He was attempting to lock eyes with me, but I was having trouble maintaining eye contact. The Expert was doing okay. I could see him and Gerry exchanging glances. *Stop talking about me with your eyes,* I wanted to shout at them. *Just get me out of here, boys. Please. Please.*

I swam out a little farther. I listened to Gerry's calm Barry White voice, but the panic would not subside. I looked at the Expert, whose eyes were wide as saucers as he watched me. Gerry looked calm, but he was starting to have trouble hiding his concern. He urged me to stop flailing my arms.

"Lay on your back," he said, "Just float. Relax."

I barrel-rolled over and floated on my back. But the pressure was worse and being on my back more closely resembled burying death by wetsuit. *Panic Number Six.* I felt the tears coming. I just floated upright and bobbed around while my goggles filled with tears. Gerry was still talking. I heard the Charlie Brown teacher in his Barry White voice. *Wah wah wah wah, I can't get enough of your love, wah wah wah, I don't know why, I can't get enough of your love, babe, wah wah wah . . .* I looked at the Expert, beseeching him with my eyes and wanting him to stop this somehow.

Screw it, I finally thought. *The longer I bob here, the longer I'm going to be stuck out here.* I looked at the boys, the buoys, and said, "I'm ready. Let's go." I had to swim, so I could get out of that water.

The three of us swam to the next buoy. And the next. And the next. I would start off okay, but then five strokes into each set, I sat up, sputtering and gasping and melting down from the fear. I was wheezing profusely. Face back in the water, swim a few strokes, feel as if I was being buried alive, then pop up again, panic, and cry. *Panics Number Seven Through Eleven.*

At the end of thirty minutes, the Expert, Gerry and I had made complete circle of the buoys, about 800 meters. At the last buoy, I turned toward shore. I doggy paddled back to the beach, the whole time praying that I would make it back to the sand before my heart exploded.

Once on land, I was dizzy.

I was deflated.

I was scared.

But I was mostly sad.

I had believed that the swim would be my thing—the best part of triathlon for me. But thanks to the blasted wetsuit, the cold water, the compression coupled with some sort of seemingly allergic reaction or a 100 percent panic attack, I felt as if I would be forced to give up triathlon.

My workout for the day was a scheduled mini-triathlon. The swim was behind me, so I decided to move on, keep my head up, and conquer the bike.

I couldn't ride. We turned back less than ten minutes after we set out. I tried to run. I ran 100 yards. *Nope.* I could not do it. I was wheezing. I could not breathe. I was done. I told the Expert to finish his run. I would not be joining him.

Gerry looked at me nonchalantly and said, "We'll walk." So, we did.

Truth be told? I was absolutely humiliated. Forget the humiliation of wearing a wetsuit, because the failure was so much worse. We walked out for some time, until we could no longer see the Expert running. Gerry talked to me, calmly. I was able to get my breathing under control. He was so compassionate, so kind to me that day. He would not let me accept my embarrassment as a final exclamation point on my triathlon dream.

He veered me in other directions. He talked through facts and details. He told me stories of his bad training and racing moments. He made me feel better. We walked back to the car, and I hugged him, apologizing.

"No need to apologize," he said, matter-of-factly. "This happens to everyone at some point during triathlon. You just got yours out of the way early. We'll get you there. You can do this."

Gerry never once told me that I would fail. He never once blinked and said, *Maybe you should take up cross-stitching.* He never gave up on me. Not once, not for a single second.

And because of him, I kept going.

All of this happened *two weeks* before the race. *Two weeks*. As the Expert drove me home, I was emotionally and physically broken. "It's okay," he said to me. "You just had a bad day. It's okay."

The day had been beautiful. I had been prepared. I had put in the effort, the training. Everything had been set up for a great day. But I completely crashed. That swim was the first time I had ever experienced a pure panic attack. I had birthed two babies. During labor, I was 90 percent certain that entire bottom half would be ripped open like a scene from a horror movie, but I was never even close to scared like that first open water swim day.

Not at first, but after a few days, I began to turn the fear I had experienced into something positive. Even though the swim experience was a slice to my heart, something in me changed that day. Five years prior, if I had encountered that kind of difficulty, I would have undoubtedly said, *F it!* I would have walked away. I would have said, *Guess I'll never be able to do an open water triathlon. Guess I'm a loser. Guess that's it. Poor me. I suck. Waaa.*

While I was panicking in the water, I battled these exact thoughts. But as the hours passed, the distance from the fear increased. The words that ran through my head were, *I can't wait to get back out to that lake and figure this out.*

Later that night, I sat on the back porch with the Expert and drove him crazy with my plans, my open water swim fixes for the next time. I talked and talked and talked through the fear. I told him, "Two weeks from today, I will finish the swim at St. Anthony's. And that's that. I may be wearing my wetsuit to the pool every night for the next two weeks, but I'm going to make it."

He listened.

"But," I repeated over and over again, "I can do this." I told the Expert over and over, "I think I can. I really think I just need another chance." I talked to myself, *You can. It was just a fear. You know you can conquer it. You can.*

He listened some more.

"You can," he said, smiling.

YOU ARE IN CHARGE

The little voice in our head that tells us "I can't" isn't really *us*. It's the totality of our experiences, our failures, the insecurities and influences in our lives. At the core of our being, we also have some really amazing stuff—badassery, strength, positivity, and more. Unfortunately, life sometimes beats the shit out of us and it's hard to *listen* to those other amazing voices. When my mind starts to tell me mean things, I like to remind it that *I* am in charge—the real me—not the one that has been beaten down. The Meredith who came into this world with everything to win and gain. That's me. And that is the voice that I choose to listen to.

Was I always this way? Hell, no. The Fat Stranger was also mean, and I spent a lot of my life hearing the "I am not good enough" voices that were projected on me from other people, then transferred to myself.

I had to work (correction: I still work) very hard to get past the negative voices, the "I can't"s and "Who do I think I am"s to make progress in life and in tri. I had to work through those even harder to get to my first triathlon. But here's the thing: if I can do it, so can you.

I am in charge of *me*. You are in charge of *you*. Remember that. The thoughts and voices in your head are *yours* to change, accept, or reject. Figure out which voices are working for your good, which ones are not so great, the ones that are downright evil, and start to categorize them as if you are having a moving sale: keep, fix, or trash.

MENTAL BADASSERY

Mental toughness is not only about the capacity to suffer. Your capacity to suffer will actually increase by training—the more you swim, bike, and run—the harder it will get, but also, paradoxically, the easier it will be to suffer, to endure, and to persevere.

Mental strength is also about maintaining the quality of your life and your goals during your triathlon training. Each day, you must utilize the greatness that is in your mind to *tell your body what it will do*. Remember, you are in charge! If you practice these principles every day, then race day just becomes an extension of your new habit. You cannot show up on race day and expect to do things you haven't done in training.

Very few people, let alone triathletes, practice mental training techniques. But, we need to practice these things for our *mind* to control our *body*—to train and to become triathletes!

GOT MANTRA?

Choosing a mantra—or the thing you will repeat when you are feeling down, suffering in a race, or doubting your abilities—is something that will serve you very well during life and tri. What will you say to yourself during training or a race when things "happen" or begin to get difficult? What will you say when your body feels as though it can't move another step? *Just keep moving forward. I got this. My body does awesome things. Keep going strong. You are strong.* It does not matter *what* you say, as long as you have something to recharge your mind and keep you focused on the goal.

During one of my races, I continually repeated: *You can stop when this is over, but you can't stop yet.* Silly, really, but it was something that made total sense to me in the moment. You can have these ready-to-use mantras in your pocket or come into them on the fly—when needed. But always have the idea of some easy, yet powerful mantra at your disposal. The power of words is magnificent!

SEE IT, BELIEVE IT.

Visualize your race as part of your training. I like to visualize not only the perfect day, but also the things that might go crazy. I don't do this to send myself into a frenzy but, rather, to keep in my mind that I am strong and I can overcome race obstacles. In this visualization, I work to remember that the only things that I can control are my attitude and my post-race snacks.

In other words, it helps to visualize yourself in a positive, focused mental state *no matter what happens* on race day. Anticipate things that could happen (e.g., choppy swim conditions, a flat tire, leg cramps on the run, etc.)—and visualize yourself dealing with all of these events with a clear, focused mind and a positive mental outlook. When things "happen," as they inevitably will, you will have worked through those issues mentally, be able to leverage your mantras to keep you going, and be ready to handle the problems. Some amazing athletes claim to have a plan, but when things go badly in a race, you can see them falling apart—they do not react well. I've seen these "thoroughbred horses" cracked into pieces on the side of the road. Then there's me, the old farm mule, just plowing through by sheer mental strength and preparation.

One of the most wonderful things about the mental side of triathlon is realizing and rediscovering that most of our limits are actually self-imposed. If the twenty-year-old me would have said, "Meredith, you will do four IRONMAN triathlons," I would have laughed. But I started. I moved forward, worked consistently on both the physical and the mental portions of training, and shattered through my self-imposed limitations.

Building mental toughness is a precious skill. Sometimes the building seems to take forever. If you are constantly growing, this is one of the skills that will take a lifetime to master. But the dividends paid are massive. Being fierce and confident is not just for eight-year-old girls—we all have that inside us. We can do it, develop it as well. I have argued so many times that mental toughness is *the* reason that I have finished so many races without quitting. When the going gets tough, I just keep going.

You have it within you to do the same.

DOUBT: THE ENEMY

When I first started training, I had to make a consistent effort to restrain myself from my typical modus operandi of self-sabotage. Even when I had completed hours of training, I would doubt my ability to race. During some of the harder months of training, I doubted my ability to do that first half Ironman—big time.

For almost a year, I had been going back and forth with a hip injury. After my first 13-mile run followed by a very long day in heels at work,

I pretty much began to hurt all the time. I was forced to admit that my pain was real, present. But I recognized that, in my usual way of self-sabotage, I might be using the pain as an *excuse* to devalue my abilities and cop out of my big race.

> "Fear is probably the thing that limits performance more than anything—the fear of not doing well, of what people will say. You've got to acknowledge those fears, then release them."
>
> —MARK ALLEN, SIX-TIME IRONMAN WORLD CHAMPION

There is advantage in the wisdom won from pain, I would tell myself, repeating one of my favorite quotes from Aeschylus.

At physical therapy during this time, the massage therapist dug into my hip and butt for trigger-point therapy. He hit one spot that immediately brought tears to my eyes, what I call the "hurts so good" factor. He said, "You are the first person in thirty years of massage therapy who didn't scream, cry, or crawl away with that point."

So, I have a high pain threshold. So what? Am I bragging? No, quite the opposite, actually.

Once I understood my high tolerance for the physical pain, I realized that my doubt issues fell somewhere in my *head*—not in my *body*. I could physically *tolerate* the pain. But the question was: could I *mentally* tolerate it? Was I mentally strong enough to make it to and through my training and the big race?

Do not let a single negative thought creep in your head during the swim or the race in general. If you feel a negative thought coming, push it out. If you are in the open water and you feel it coming, then sing a song, breaststroke, but do not let negativity in.

You might ask, "Well, what if I am panicking?"

The answer is: no no no. Do not even *utter* words like *panic* and *fear*. Knock them out of your head now, in the beginning and in training, and while you are on the land. And do not let them return.

When the doubt comes in, push it away. Pretend you are a cat and you are playing with a crazy cat toy called Doubt. Bat that shit away over and over until you can bat it no more. Then bat it again. Get the doubt away from you—no matter what it takes.

JUST SHOW UP

In the book *Your First Triathlon*, triathlon coach Joe Friel writes about the importance of never skipping scheduled training days. He emphasizes that the level of commitment to triathlon must be hard-core. I totally agree, and I also agree with another point of his: if you commit to getting dressed and giving your workout a promised five minutes, chances are, you will finish the workout. Then, if after five minutes, you cannot do it, stop moving, give up, because today is *not* your day. Just do better tomorrow.[1]

I have found the five-minute rule to be fairly true. If I make the effort to wake up early, get dressed, and drive to the gym, and I am a complete crabapple, usually I will snap out of my funk after five minutes. I may not be singing songs and skipping happy while I complete the workout, but usually I can scrounge up enough fortitude to finish.

However, I have stumbled across a handful of days, outside of being sick, where I did not feel like running, jogging, walking, cycling (indoors or outdoors), swimming, or floating. Days where I just wanted to be lazy for no apparent reason. But I always tried my best to *never* skip a scheduled workout. Even feeling like garbage, I would get dressed, strap on the heart rate monitor, the shoes, or the swimsuit. But only a few times, I jogged or swam for five minutes and actually threw in the towel.

The best thing to remember is that walking away from the workout is sometimes okay. You made the effort to show up, you put in the attempt, and if it does not happen that day, forget about it and move on. When that happens, I say to myself: *I will do better tomorrow. That's all I can do for today.*

FOCUSING ON WHAT YOU CAN DO

I am not one to throw in the proverbial towel when things get difficult. Not externally, I should add. I rarely throw my hands up, scream "I quit," and walk away. Instead, I tend to *internally* self-destruct. Stress at work, sick kids, and suddenly, I find myself eating a pint of ice cream in the closet and listening to *Boys for Pele* underneath my old prom dresses. Once the pint is scraped clean and a few rounds of "Hey Jupiter" have flashed through my head, I am back to business as usual. Only the "business" is planted firmly on my rear end in the form of fat cells and regret.

About ten weeks to my first Olympic distance race, I was awake all night with a sick baby. My alarm was set for 4:30 a.m. to wake up for cycling class. Mistakenly, however, I had set the alarm for p.m. Needless to say, cycling class happened 30 miles away that morning without me. I knew that the one instance was just a boo-boo, a mistake, and a life happening. I needed to stay home anyway, because the kid was sick.

But the question for the rest of the day was how to deal mentally and emotionally with a missed workout, sleep deprivation, a ton of work to accomplish and no way to do it because of caring for a sick child? The tougher question was how to do all of that without sabotaging my diet, turning completely evil, and making excuses in perpetuity.

I started some positive self-talk. *Sure, I missed cycling class, but I own a bike in the garage. I can cycle tonight on the trainer after I tuck the kids away. Sure, coach won't be yelling at me from the seat, motivating me, but it's something.*

As for the food and the sabotage, I created another dialogue. *Yes, I am home today. But I don't freaking live in a Taco Bell. I can control my diet.*

And finally: *I have a computer and a babysitter who will come in for a few hours. I can work from home, breaking only to eat (not at the Taco Bell) and take the baby to the doctor. That kills two birds with one stone: being a conscientious employee and a "decent" mother.*

That small positive self-talk movement was the beginning of focusing on what I *could* do, instead of getting hung up on what I couldn't do.

As in life, so in tri. *I am defining my own life. Me. I will make my life happen. I will create the life I want.*

BOTHERSOME HAPPINESS

After almost a year of training, I found myself pretty darn happy. Interestingly, my happiness actually bothered some people. And the longer I am in this, the more I find this to still be true. *Your* happiness and strength may begin to grate on people—granted, those people might not be the type of folks you need on your side, anyway, but . . .

You must learn to keep out the bad energy. People might be annoyed by your newfound triathlon happiness. If you have not experienced the jealousy yet, you will. Friends that were "best" friends can become borderline enemies because of their bitter sarcasm directed at your journey. Just be prepared for it. Remember: your bothersome happiness is worth the ridicule.

SELF-MOTIVATION

Sometimes the hardest part about triathlon is moving forward when you are training alone. There will be times when you are the only spinner in the room, there is no music, and it's 4:30 a.m. You may be the only runner on the path (be safe). Or the lonely fish in the pool. You may be the only human for (what seems like) 100 square miles.

If triathlon teaches you anything, it will be self-motivation. At the end of the day, each training session is up to you. You have the choice to push through or ship out. Keep moving forward. Every piece of food (good or bad) that you put into your mouth is your choice. Every "snoozed" second you sleep in . . . you got it—your choice (and sometimes, the snooze button *is* the better option).

Your life is *yours*. Training by yourself is a good correlation to life in general. Start believing in yourself. Rely on yourself. Make yourself stronger. You can do it.

MENTAL TOUGHNESS: NOT JUST FOR THE PROS

Until triathlon, I had always been the type of person to focus on my weaknesses, to let my head drop. For years and years, it was all about what I could *not* do. *I can't run. I can't bike. I can't clip out of my bike pedals without falling.*

I still battle the instinct to respond to almost everything with a negative light from the get-go. Maybe it's the lawyer in me talking (*We're all going to get sued in the end, so what does it matter?*). Usually, I can turn lemons into a fabulous lemon soufflé by the *end* of the day. But my gut reaction in the morning is to scream: "Sky. Falling! See it?"

Chrissie Wellington wrote an amazing article for CNN in February 2012.[2] If you do not know about Chrissie Wellington, then you should swim, bike, and run to the video of the 2008 IRONMAN World Championship (YouTube.com has a version). Chrissie got a flat tube on the cycling leg, wasted her CO_2 cartridge, and yet, still went on for the win. She's won the IRONMAN World Championship four times and has never (ever) lost an IRONMAN distance race that she's entered. On my podcast, she recounted why she retired after her 2011 Kona appearance—citing that as her hardest yet most glorious race. She had a bike crash right before the race, her body hurt and wounded from road rash. She went into that race in pain and came out a champion once again. She went out on the highest note of her career.

One of the best quotes in the article is also one of my all-time favorites: "If we let our head drop, our heart drops with it. Keep your head up, and your body is capable of amazing feats." She also wrote that when negative thoughts arise, we must "deliver these negative thoughts a knockout punch before they have the chance to grow and become the mental monster that derails your entire race."[3] Of course, this applies to training and life, too.

The negative game I was (and sometimes am) playing is a mental beast, just as Chrissie points out. With my Decision, I decided that I would not spend so much time sitting. Then, I entered races and set goals. If only I had spent the last ten years saying, "Yes, I can do that" or "I will sure as hell try," who knows where I would be. Probably still in the back of the triathlon pack, but I would have been more calm, happy, and focused during those years—instead of stressed and hopeless.

On those long runs where I swear to my dear sweet Lord that I am about to die, I hear my brain say to my body: *You aren't going to die. The pain will stop when you stop. Just run through the pain. When you're done running, the pain will stop. But if you stop before you are done, the physical pain will become shame pain and you will have to tell your coach that you quit because "it was hard." For shame.*

Of course, along the way I experienced moments where I stomped my feet, cursed, and said, "I quit!" But overall, I maintained some form of mental toughness, even when my body was not tough, but just a flabby ball of mess.

Do not kid yourself. While vital for the pros and elite triathletes, mental toughness is even more important for the *newbies* to the sport. If you are starting out anything like I did, then you are accustomed to society (and yourself) telling you that you aren't good, pretty, thin, smart, rich, or fit *enough*. Therefore, when you make a crazy declaration like "I'm going to become a triathlete," and those same people who thought you were *fat* now think you are fat *and* crazy, your mental toughness is forced to either rise up or eat crow.

(I've never cared for crow.)

Whatever your goal, be a mental giant! Channel Chrissie Wellington. Channel the cold beer at the end of the race. Who cares how you build the toughness; just build it. Talk down those fears from the ledge in your mind. You can do it. Make it happen. No matter your size or shape, 90 percent of the people in your life won't be able to keep up . . . and they sure as hell won't know what to say when you reach your goals.

11

NUTRITION AND THE SCALE

WEIGHT HAS BEEN A LIFELONG BATTLE FOR ME. I SAT ON THE sidelines for a lot of my adult life because I was "too big," "too fat," or "too slow." Once I decided that I wouldn't wait any longer— for whatever "thinness" I needed to happen, things changed. Once I realized that as much as I tried, I *could not* be defined by the damn scale—or I would never get anywhere.

Regardless of what we weigh right now, we must move forward and work toward our health, wellness, or triathlon goals *at whatever current weight* we are. I must start now. You must start *now*.

FOOD. A LOVE STORY.

If there is a chapter in my book that I am completely incapable of writing on my own, it would be one on nutrition. Weight, dieting, nutrition, the scale, my muffin top, and self-esteem are all my sore spots. Regardless of my progress and certifications, I am a passenger on the perpetual struggle bus with food.

I will always want to weigh less than I do. I will never be content as the "bigger" version of me, just because of the way I feel when I am at a lower weight—I feel better in my own skin. No amount of self-love, acceptance, and cheerleading will cure this constant search for food and nutrition improvement for me. I know that.

But I am also realistic.

I do not say, *Oh, I can't lose weight.* Do you know why? Because I also *know* that I have not made the necessary sacrifices to have my dream bod. Have I given up pizza? *Nope.* Ice cream? *When hell freezes over.* Chocolate? *You must be kidding.*

Regardless of what you weigh right now, you must move forward and work toward your triathlon goals *at your current weight*. You must start *now*. Do *not* wait until you are "smaller" to start moving. Do not say, "When I lose weight, then I will run." That does not work, and if you are like me, you might be waiting forever!

> **D**on't Weight . . . er, Wait!
> Get moving now, at your current size! Do not wait for the perfect day, your perfect size, or perfect weather. All of these things will never happen at the same time, and you'll be waiting forever to get started. Go now!

I would have wasted the past decade if I waited to be a size 10 to run. Because just now, over eight years later, I am a size 10. I would still be waiting.

Translation: go, go, go!

JUST KEEP TRYING

One of the things I have realized is most effective with weight and nutrition is simply a level of consistency. Not perfection, just continuing to try to improve yourself from a health standpoint. No matter what the scale says or society says—the question to ask is: how can I *feel* my best?

When you fail, you pick up and keep going. You never give up on *you*. Sometimes you get it right, and sometimes you eat the "egg yellows." I explain.

After a Friday morning cycling class, I went to a fast-food joint for a quick breakfast. I knew it was a bad idea, but I was in a hurry, having failed to prepare.

I pulled up to the drive-through, rolled down my window, and ordered something very reasonable: a plain breakfast wrap with egg and coffee. I asked if they had salsa (they did not). I reminded them that I did not want cheese or anything else (they understood).

"A plain egg wrap, no cheese. A large coffee," I said into the speaker.

"Do you want bacon?"

"No," I said, "Please, no bacon. Just plain egg and wrap. Actually, do you have egg whites?" (This was before I learned the whole egg was great.)

"Who?"

"What?" I asked.

"Egg who?" the speaker asked.

"Egg whites, do you—"

"—no, we only got egg yellows."

"Egg yellows?"

"Yeah."

I stared at the speaker. *Egg yellows?*

"All right. Just yellow eggs and a wrap. Thanks."

"Drive around."

As I drove down the road with my decently healthy food sitting in a brown bag in the seat beside me, I felt proud of myself. Proud that I did not give in to the Fat Stranger screaming: *Get the bacon, cheese biscuit! Oh, and a cinnamon roll! Two cinnamon rolls!*

So, I was on a bit of a high from Spin class, feeling proud from ordering healthy and I thought I was ready to tackle my day. As I opened my little healthy breakfast on the highway, I gasped.

I was clutching a steaming hot wrap filed with egg, all right.

But it was *also* boiling over with sausage, cheese, and (wait for it . . . wait for it . . .) hash browns. Hash brown potatoes, snuggled up to the sausage and cheese. I cursed out loud and hit my steering wheel.

Dammit! I tried to do the right thing! I tried! I tried to be healthy! And this! *This?!* I was so mad. So mad.

So, I ate it.

KEEPING TRACK OF WHAT I PUT IN MY MOUTH

Triathlon has done amazing things for my body over the last almost-decade. Regardless, I continue to battle the bulge. Getting older doesn't help this, either. Part of my weight struggle has been simple overeating, but I have also spent decades battling binge eating to the point of disorder. Bingeing is bad news and can really mess with your heart, soul, and body. Obviously, eating disorders are well beyond the scope of this book, but I do highly recommend *Brain Over Binge* as a resource for anyone who might be experiencing eating disorders.

Over the years, I have learned that simply shifting my thoughts from *weight loss* to *health* has changed most for me in the world of weight.

If I am just thinking, *What will make me* feel *best?* I tend to eat well, take care of myself, and binge less. If I think about health, then I am more inclined to be kinder to myself. Kindness is everything.

Focusing also on the greatness that my body *is* has shifted the focus from appearance to movement. *Look how flexible I can be. Look how hard I will work, how much I will sweat.* Taking stock of how far we have come—even if the scale doesn't budge—there are victories everywhere.

I try to keep track of what I put in my mouth. To log it, to eat *mindfully* and not as if I am starving. I realized that because I was force-dieted as a kid, that I fear feeling hungry. Addressing those feelings and recognizing that feeling hungry is okay sometimes—and sitting with those emotions—is an important part of my relationship with food journey.

Finally, if you like to have data, I would implore you to take out your tape measure instead of your scale. While I often do not have drastic reduction of measurements in the obvious places—hips and stomach—in recent years I have lost over 2 1/2 *inches* off my neck, of all places. I had no idea my neck was storing flubber. Now, I take great joy in my neck. It's important to find these small joys and victories in our journeys.

NUTRITION AND TRIATHLON NUTRITION
FOR THE EVERY WOMAN

Dina Griffin, MS, RDN, CSSD, CISSN
www.NutritionMechanic.com

I met Dina Griffin in very early 2017 when I started learning about the impor-
tance of balancing blood sugar so as to use some of my plentiful body fat for fuel.
With her help, I jump-started some year-long stagnation and learned to take my
body composition to leaner places. I adore Dina for her authentic personality,
her unparalleled years of true expertise, and the way that she cares for her cli-
ents. Not only that, but Dina is an endurance athlete and a true genius when
it comes to endurance and racing fueling. There is truly no one better to write
about nutrition for the "Every Woman" than this amazing lady! Here's Dina:

The beauty of females, particularly female athletes, is that we are
unique. We each have "nutrition subtleties" to learn and master for our
optimum health, longevity, and athletic performance. In other words,
two female triathletes who are similar in age, physical characteristics,
and exercise patterns may require completely different nutrition patterns
to achieve their unique optimum. Why? Factors such as hormonal balance, coexisting medical conditions, genetics, and athletic ability contribute more to our nutritional needs than we might believe!

On top of that, what we actually *like* to eat versus what we *should*
eat to support our health and training goals can be tricky. Decoding all
of these factors can be frustrating, but as Meredith says—forward is a
pace—and patience with the entire process of triathlon training *and* nutrition is a must. As a registered dietitian, board-certified sport dietitian,
and one who works with all levels of recreational and competitive triathletes, I have seen it all when it comes to nutrition and food patterns—
one of the reasons I love what I do!

A quick backstory about me. I became a triathlete at the ripe age of
thirty-four, a few years before I became a dietitian. I started like many
other female triathletes—no athletic background as a youth, with only

a few years of adult-onset exercise. In my first triathlon sprint race, I self-seeded in the "beginner" wave due to race anxiety and fear of getting trampled in the swim. Long story short, it turned out to be an incredibly memorable, fun, and life-changing experience. Several years later, and many triathlon finish lines crossed (including the IRONMAN distance), it is a sport I will forever love.

In my growth as an endurance athlete and in my work as a sport dietitian having supported hundreds of female triathletes over the years, I can say truthfully that nutrition—both daily and race day—can make or break your race. It sounds harsh and dramatic, I know. But getting a sour stomach or the "Porta-Potty tour" due to poor race day nutrition planning and implementation is no fun and can take away from all of the hard work you put into your training. Additionally, daily nutrition is the key foundational element to your training and racing more so than what you nibble on during a workout.

Before we get into more nutrition nitty gritty, here are my Every Woman nutrition tenets to help you on your journey.

Beware of the Comparison and Data Craze

As Meredith alludes to earlier, comparing your triathlon goals to others' can be big trouble. Same goes for your "nutrition lifestyle" and your health goals. Far too many times have I heard women compare their eating to men, their BFFs, or their work colleagues. Even within our own life span, we may find that the nutrition pattern that worked earlier in life no longer works at another point in life. *You* and your food lifestyle are unique to *you*, so aim to stay true to yourself and live (and adjust) in the moment and forward.

As much as many of us live by numbers and data, such as daily steps taken, average pace for a run or miles per hour on the bike, calorie counts, macronutrient counts, how many ounces of water we drink in a day, and the number on the weight scale, numerous factors affect our food choices. It's okay to have objective motivators that are numbers-oriented, but numbers are not the be-and-end-all. Let yourself *feel* the effects of your food choices and *reflect* on how they are working (or not) for you, so that you'll know better when it is time for change.

If you would like to lose weight, a few points. Remember: you are *not* defined by the diet or dietary pattern you follow. Just as the number on the scale does not define you, nor does the width of your hips, your shoe size, or the length of your pinkie finger, the food pattern you follow is not *you*. Why do I mention this? Truly, with the hoopla of Internet forums and social media groups, it is easy to fall into nutrition dogma or even become so emotionally wrapped up in a "my way or the highway" diet cult following. It truly is important to remember that you are far more than your body weight and the number on the scale. The way you look shouldn't rule your existence. Remember that the goal of this triathlon journey is to better your life. Sure, weight loss might be a part of the journey and it also might be necessary. But try to shift away from that focus for a bit. Think about what your body *can* do right now. Start with health and how you feel—work on that, and let food be the fuel for your amazing machine. With health comes . . . well, health! And that is truly what you are seeking.

Daily Nutrition

Although you may think focusing on race nutrition (or what you can eat since you worked so hard) is the key, it's daily nutrition that is the foundation of your health and your triathlon abilities.

In fact, look at the many areas in which daily nutrition can affect your existence:

- Body composition
- Energy levels
- Mood
- Cognition
- Workout recoveries

- Hormonal balance
- Sleep quality
- Immune system health
- Disease prevention

To name a few. And while not all of these may seem directly related to you, a triathlete, they can absolutely affect your training and longevity in the sport.

So, here's the question: which dietary pattern is best for you?

The answer is: it depends!

As mentioned earlier, because each of us is unique in terms of our body (metabolism, hormones, physiology) and brain (emotions, coping, stress, habits), each of us must find our own way. In light of this, I want to provide core concepts and tips that you can digest (see what I did there?) and apply to your current food lifestyle. You may not buy into all of these tips right away, so go ahead and revisit this chapter when you're ready for things to sink in. Once you grasp these concepts, you become freer in your nutrition journey going forward!

Disclaimer: If you are on a medically supervised diet or a specific clini-cally prescribed dietary plan, please consult with your doctor before making any changes.

Make Protein a Priority

Protein does wonders for health and supporting your training, no mat-ter what dietary pattern you follow—plant-based, omnivore, or hard-core carnivore. Dietary protein plays a role in aspects we should care about, including immune system health, bone and soft tissue health, wound healing, and muscle growth and repair.

One of the extra-special fun facts about protein is that it helps keep you full—or as we dietitians say, you achieve satiety. You can test this easily for yourself. Choose a food, such as an apple or some carrots. Eat this as a snack and notice how long it takes until you start to feel the nosh-nosh urge coming on. The next day at the same time, repeat this experiment, but include a source of protein. Notice that you feel fuller for a longer period of time? Yeaaah. Protein is the real deal.

Particularly for female triathletes, protein is not a macronutrient to skimp on. Even if you desire to lose weight while training, higher protein intake not only serves to keep you full for a longer period of time, but consuming more protein can help with gain (or maintenance) of lean muscle tissue, especially if strength or resistance work is incorporated into a training regimen.

Reference the following list of protein sources and think about your current intake. Ask yourself these questions: *Can I add more types of proteins? Does each meal I eat contain one or more proteins?*

Examples of Plant Protein Sources			
Adzuki beans	Edamame/soy-beans	Mung beans	Pumpkin seeds
Almonds	Fava beans	Natto	Quinoa (or whole grains for vegans)
Black beans	Fortified nondairy milks	Nut/seed butters	Sacha Inchi seeds
Brazil nuts	Hemp	Pecans	Sunflower seeds
Cashews	Kidney beans	Pinto beans	Tempeh
Chia	Lentils	Pistachio nuts	Tofu
Chickpeas	Macadamia nuts	Plant-based protein powder	Walnuts
Examples of Animal Protein Sources			
Bacon	Chicken	Pork	Shellfish
Beef	Cottage cheese	Protein powder (beef, egg, whey, casein)	Turkey
Bison	Eggs/egg whites	Sausage	Wild game
Cheese	Milk (cow or goat)	Seafood	Yogurt (cow or goat)

Protein Tips for the Every Woman Triathlete

- As a triathlete, you can be more lenient in your protein amounts so long as you are choosing quality protein sources. Gone are the days when you were strictly limited to a tiny, palm-size amount of protein at each meal (3 ounces by weight). Instead, include 4 to 6 ounces of protein at each meal (or 25–40 grams by content; closer to two palms!).
- It is well established that as we age (past age 35!), we start losing muscle mass. Staying physically fit with routine weight lifting can help mitigate this, but eating 25 to 40 grams of protein at each meal throughout the day has a significant impact on lessening lean muscle loss throughout our latter decades of life.
- If it is within your budget and you eat animal protein, aim to include grass-fed meats, wild-caught fish, pasture-raised poultry, organic dairy, and wild game as often as you can for a better nutritional profile.
- If you follow vegetarian or vegan patterns, be mindful of your intake of processed foods (e.g., veggie burgers/cheeses/hot dogs/etc.). Whole food, plant-based proteins will serve your body better than will highly processed protein sources.

Fat Phobia, Be Gone!

Depending on your age and dieting background, dietary fat may evoke images of food horror and evil in your mind. *Egads, the stick of butter will stick to my hips if I even give it a glance!*

Take a deep breath and check this out: fats are back. They never went away, actually. But they were given the stink eye for a few too many decades.

You *need* fats for many critical functions in the body, including absorption of fat-soluble vitamins (A, D, E, K), hormonal regulation, in addition to maintaining brain and nervous system health. An effect you may actually "feel" from eating fats is that we stay full for a longer period of time. Hey, that's something in common with eating protein—increased satiety!

Fats are also a good energy source, giving us more than twice the calories per gram than proteins and carbohydrates can. You may know already know that fact and cringe, thinking, *fats are evil—they make me fat!*

We won't gain body fat by the mere act of eating dietary fat. It is more complicated than that. For example, do you have a good awareness of your biological level of hunger and fullness to know how much to eat or when to stop eating? Do you eat slowly? Do you eat with intention or are you mindlessly grazing? What else is in the meal, besides fat (e.g., is it a greasy burger with fries and a milk shake or a salmon fillet with olive oil–drizzled broccoli and an almond rice pilaf)?

The fact is, weight gain can happen if we overeat *any* type of calories, not just from fat sources. However, knowing that protein and fat-containing foods are the "sustainers" and that the majority of female athletes tend to underconsume these sticking-power foods, it begs the case for giving a fresh look at your intake at *each* meal.

Examples of Plant-Derived Fat Sources			
Avocados	Coconut milk	Hummus	Olive oil
Avocado oil	Coconut oil	MCT oil	Palm oil
Chia	Flax meal	Nuts/nut butters	Seeds/seed butters
Coconut butter	Flax oil	Nut-based milks	Tempeh/tofu
Coconut flakes	Hemp hearts	Olives	Walnut oil
Examples of Animal-Derived Fat Sources			
Butter/ghee	Cream cheese (fuller fat)	Half-and-half	Sausage
Cottage cheese (fuller fat)	Egg yolks	Higher-fat meats/ poultry	Tallow
Cream	Fattier fish and their oils (salmon, sardines, anchovies, cod liver oil)	Milk (fuller fat; cow or goat)	Yogurt (fuller fat; cow or goat)

Fat Tips for the Every Woman Triathlete

- Aim for variety and quality in your fat-containing foods.
  - » You probably need to include more plant-derived sources of fats and increase your intake of omega-3 fats and monounsaturated fats. To do this, include more avocado, raw walnuts and other raw nuts, flax, olives and their oils. If you eat fish, go for more salmon, trout, and sardines.
  - » Reduce or minimize your intake of fried foods or classic baked goods (calling all doughnut lovers!). By doing so, you lessen the impact of highly processed fats (including *trans* fats) on your body, which suits your health goals and helps you for the long haul!
  - » If you are a meat and dairy lover, look for ways to include plant sources of fats in your meals. Swap out a higher-animal-fat food for a plant-based-fat food. For example, drizzle olive oil on your salads or cooked vegetables, include a side of sliced avocado, or add toasted pumpkin seeds or walnuts to your salads instead of bacon bits, cheese chunks, or the heavy drizzle of blue cheese dressing.
  - » Vegans and vegetarians tend to consume a low-fat diet. Experiment with adding more fats and see how you feel.
  - » When choosing animal- or marine-derived fats, it is ideal to choose wild-caught fish (or sustainably raised from trusted sources), grass-fed meats or wild game, and pasture-raised poultry, if it fits within your budget, to get a better fatty acid profile.
- Be mindful of portion sizes. We can be "healthy eaters" and still overeat if we aren't being reasonable with food amounts, particularly when fats are present in meals and snacks.

Strategy and Selectivity with Carbohydrates

First of all, *carbs are not bad*. I am not here to tell you, "No carbs for you, Every Woman Triathlete!" Contrary to popular thinking, you can still eat carb-containing foods and make progress in your journey to become the triathlete you want to be!

The issue is that many women athletes generally fall into one of these categories:

1. We are eating *types* of carbohydrates that don't serve our body well, from a health perspective and/or from an athletic perspective. Our *selectivity* may need improvement.
2. We eat an inappropriate *amount* of carbs (which could be on either end of the spectrum—too little or too much). Our *strategy* for carb consumption may need to be examined.
3. A mix of both #1 and #2—shucks.

How do you address this? First, remember that you are not looking to go on the D3 (dreaded deprivation diet). Get your mind-set into the "How do I eat more optimally for *my* health goals and *my* triathlete goals?"

Carbohydrate foods fall into these basic categories: vegetables, fruits, legumes, whole grains, processed/refined carbs, and added sugars. However, carbs are also contained in such foods as yogurt, milk (cow/goat/soy), nuts, and seeds.

For daily nutrition, the emphasis should be on *a variety of whole food, fiber-rich, nutrient-dense sources of carbohydrates*. That is: vegetables, fruits, legumes, and whole grains. When you look really closely at what you eat in a given day, you may be surprised to see a lack of vegetables and a reliance on processed carbs.

Carbohydrates are way more than "energy foods." If you choose the right (or the better) kinds of carb-containing foods, then you reap the benefits of fiber (which you need for gut health and to help keep you feeling full), micronutrients (vitamins and minerals), and phytonutrients (other plant-derived compounds that have protective health benefits).

Check out the following table for ideas and reminders of foods that fall into the quality-carbohydrate categories. Note that these food groupings are based on a nutritional context, not a botanical one. For example, tomatoes are technically classified as a fruit, but here they are in the vegetable category based on their carbohydrate characteristics.

Examples of Vegetables			
Artichoke	Cauliflower	Kohlrabi	Rutabaga
Arugula	Chard	Leeks	Snap peas
Asparagus	Collard greens	Mushrooms	Spinach
Beets	Endive	Mustard greens	Squashes
Bell peppers	Eggplants	Okra	Sweet potatoes
Bok choy	Fennel	Onions	Tomatoes
Broccoli	Green beans	Parsnips	Turnip
Brussels sprouts	Jicama	Radicchio	Water chestnuts
Cabbage	Kale	Radish	Watercress
Carrots	Kimchi	Rhubarb	Zucchini

Examples of Fruits			
Apples	Cherries	Grapes	Pears
Apricots	Dates	Kiwis	Plantains
Bananas	Dragon fruit	Mangoes	Plums
Blackberries	Figs	Nectarines	Pomegranates
Blueberries	Goji berries	Oranges	Raspberries
Cantaloupe	Grapefruit	Peaches	Strawberries

Examples of Whole Grains			
Amaranth*	Einkorn	Millet*	Sorghum*
Barley	Farro	Oats**	Spelt
Buckwheat*	Freekeh	Quinoa*	Teff*
Bulgur	Kamut	Rice*	Triticale
Corn*	Kaniwa*	Rye	Wheat

*gluten-free; **typically gluten-free, but check packaging if you need to be gluten-free

Now take a preview of some of the common carbohydrates that are processed and refined, or items that contain added sugar.

Examples of Processed/Refined Carbs and Added Sugars			
Agave	Crackers	Muffins	Wine
Breads	Honey	Ice cream	Liquor
Candy	Table sugar	Frozen yogurt	Maple syrup
Chips	Sweetened tea	Sorbet	Chocolate
Cookies	Mocha coffee	Beer	Pretzels

You can quickly detect the difference in food quality between the two sets of tables. Again, it doesn't mean you should never, ever, evvaaahhh eat or drink anything that is processed, refined, or contains added sugar. It just means that 80 to 90 percent of your everyday eating should be focused on the "better for you" carbohydrate foods.

How do you know how much carbohydrate to eat? That, my friends, is a great question and one best answered with, once again, "It depends!" (sorry to say). Because everyone is unique, some people can tolerate a large amount of carbohydrates with no problem, while others cannot due to medical conditions (such as diabetes, insulin resistance, or polycystic ovarian syndrome), gene variants, or behavior related issues that contribute to overeating of hyperpalatable sugary foods. Additionally, depending on the workouts planned for the day, there may or may not be a need for increased carbohydrate consumption.

Carbohydrate Tips for the Every Woman Triathlete

- If you desire fat loss, focus on getting the majority of your carbohydrate intake from vegetables. If most of your vegetables are starchy in nature (e.g., peas, corn, potatoes) and you haven't seen progress with your weight loss, then incorporate more nonstarchy vegetables. Moderate your fruit and grain intake, or try minimizing these foods on sedentary or less physically active days. Be mindful of your intake of sweets, alcohol, and processed/refined carbs.
- The female body stores 1,200 to 1,500 carbohydrate calories on average. For days involving 60 to 90 minutes or less of exercise, you don't need to add gobs of simple sugars to your day to fuel the workout. Your body has internal carb sources to help you out! Start training your body to be less dependent on simple sugars for those shorter workouts and don't overfeed it.
- For keeping you full longer and stabilizing your blood sugar levels (which has many metabolic benefits), always pair a carbohydrate food with one or more sources of protein and/or fat. For example,

instead of snacking on the apple by itself, include some nuts, a piece of cheese, Greek yogurt, or some hummus.

- Remember quality. You can actually eat quite a lot of vegetables and other whole food–based carbs and get far more nutritional benefit than you will from the same number of calories from a processed grain.
- If you are a self-proclaimed picky eater when it comes to vegetables, you owe it to yourself to experiment and have a fresh start away from any childhood memories that linger. Try vegetables prepared differently, such as by roasting or grilling. Try new seasonings, salsas, hot sauces, or infused olive oils. There are lots of new flavors for you to discover!
- Even changing one high-carb, low-nutrient-dense snack or meal *each day* can make a difference. For example, replace dried fruit with fresh fruit. Trade the hoagie bread for lettuce wraps or eat only half of the bread. Replace the soda and chips with a seltzer water, salted veggies, and dip.
- Do an inventory of your "go-to" carbs and give them a fresh eye. It's likely that you have a good sense of whether your selection and eating pattern of carbohydrate-containing foods need some improvement. It's never too late to make positive changes!

Life Is Hard. Food Doesn't Have to Be.

As you hopefully know now (via the broken record playing repeatedly), there is no single diet, calorie count, or macronutrient profile that will work for everyone. If you grimace and grunt when hearing that statement (or the often quoted "Find what works for you!"), try to reframe your mind-set.

If you have been stuck and on your own, it's okay to reach out to a sport dietitian or other qualified health professional for guidance as you start this li'l (big) thing called triathlon training. Just like hiring a coach for your training, a swim instructor to figure out how to do more than doggy paddle swim, or the bike mechanic to fix the "what's this here part called?" professional nutrition guidance can do wonders for assessing your needs and outlining a plan specific to you.

Food is powerful. Your body is complex, but fueling it in positive and sustaining ways does not have to be complicated. As a female triathlete, you owe it to yourself to nourish your body to support your special health and your triathlon journey.

Daily Hydration

Proper hydration has many functions within the body to keep it running at maximum efficiency. These functions include:

- Aiding in digestion and absorption of nutrients
- Filtering and elimination of waste products (yep, sweat, urine, and . . .)
- Bowel regularity
- Protection and growth of skin
- Support of exercise performance by reducing body organ strain (heart, skin, muscles, nervous system, kidneys) and regulating core temperature
- Reduction of risk for bladder infections, kidney stones, and compromised respiratory function

Unfortunately, hydration is often neglected until it's too late. Perhaps you know the feeling. A sudden overwhelming sense of thirst later in the day necessitating an immediate need to guzzle the Big Gulp–size water bottle. Or the afternoon "brain fuzz" or mild headache when you suddenly realize you've ignored drinking any fluids except for your morning starter coffee. The Hurry Up and Hydrate approach doesn't really work quickly, though, so caution must be heeded.

While a bunch of formulas are out there to guide you in how much you should drink each day, none of them is foolproof. For example, a common guideline is to drink half of your body weight (in pounds) in water (in ounces) each day. While this may be a decent starting point, the guideline doesn't consider other factors that can influence fluid needs, such as activity level or type of exercise day, environmental conditions (e.g., hot/humid vs. colder/drier), sweat rates, pregnancy or postpartum status, and water content from consumed foods (e.g., fruits and vegetables). Of course, you can use formulas as a guideline, but it is important to gauge how you feel and experiment with your fluid intake to determine your "hydration sweet spot."

Although plain water can certainly comprise a good portion of your daily fluid intake, your body benefits from many types of fluids. I'm not talking the extra-large soda or the ginormous sweetened tea (you don't need all of those added sugars!). Rather, seltzer and mineral waters, unsweetened milks (dairy or nondairy), smoothies, vegetable and fruit juices (though you need to be mindful of the carbohydrate load from fruit juices), kombucha, and broths or soups. Consuming a variety of vegetables and fruits also provides your body with some fluid from their respective water content. Think: lettuces and leafy greens, bell peppers, tomatoes, cucumbers, melons, berries, or other juicy vegetables and fruits.

Should you consume sweetened beverages if it helps you drink more fluids? The short answer is no. Highly concentrated sugar-laden drinks can actually *de*hydrate you. And in the Mrs. Obvious department, the added sugar calories offer nothing beneficial to body composition goals (unless you are looking to gain weight), systemic inflammation, or reduction of any carboholic-sugar tendencies.

So, should you just park yourself by the garden hose? Nope. Guzzling copious amounts of plain water, especially when exercising, can lower your blood sodium concentration, resulting in a range of side effects (from dizziness, muscle weakness, and nausea to the more extreme outcomes of coma or death due to brain swelling). Additionally, you actually won't hydrate very well if you rely exclusively on lots of plain water for your exercise days, particularly in hot and/or humid weather conditions. In essence, your body won't "hold on to" plain water, so you end up peeing it out more than absorbing it. You can mitigate this by either drinking only moderate amounts of water, by adding sodium to your water (even just a pinch of table salt), or by incorporating foods or other beverages that contain salt (sodium).

Did I mention alcohol? You don't want to rely on the salted rim of the margarita to get your extra sodium, nor do you want to let alcoholic beverages get in the way of your daily hydration or preparation for workouts. I'm not saying you should never have an alcoholic beverage while you live your triathlon life. If you can control and moderate your alcohol consumption, then it may fit in your lifestyle. However, it does not play a role in "proper" hydration.

As far as knowing how to determine whether you are well hydrated, there really isn't a perfect method unless you are in a hospital being monitored by a doctor. Generally, you can pay attention to your pee frequency (is it every few hours vs. only a few times per day), urine color (while there are various influences, in general, a lighter color means better hydration), and your sense of thirst (although this changes with age!). A rule of thumb is to drink when you feel thirsty, but be proactive and don't let yourself get in the thirst danger zone. Have some common sense and remember the importance of hydration for daily living and to support your tri training.

Hydration Tips for the Every Woman

- If you struggle with drinking plain water, remember you can expand your beverage choices while including more vegetables and fruits.
- Don't rely on sports drinks for your daily hydration. There is a time and a place for sports drinks. And not all are created the same or serve your body well for daily hydration or for exercise hydration.
- Although hotly debated among those in the health community, beverages containing artificial sweeteners, such as aspartame and sucralose, won't dehydrate you per se. The concern is more whether these ingredients are "needed" and their potential impact on appetite, the brain reward center, and hormonal regulation.

- Caffeinated beverages also won't dehydrate you. Caffeine can make you pee more often, but research has demonstrated that moderate caffeine intake is not a dehydrator on its own.
- Examine all of your fluid sources carefully and then pick your battles. For example, if you are reliant on mostly diet sodas or sweetened coffee drinks for most of your fluid intake during the day, then you can start a weaning process. Consider replacing each diet soda with a flavored unsweetened bubbly or decrease the size of the sweetened coffee drink and order it with half the goodies. You don't have to go cold turkey to make positive changes.

Hydration for Training

Sweat is no longer a four-letter word. For the recommended amount of fluid to drink during exercise, it depends on what type of exercise you are doing, the duration, the intensity, and how much you sweat. A general range is 16 to 32 ounces per hour, but that's a pretty big range! For you to better know how much fluid you should be drinking, it behooves you to learn your sweat rate and monitor it periodically throughout your training. Sweat rate, simply defined, is how much sweat your body generates. It is usually reported in ounces or milliliters per hour.

Be aware that your sweat rate changes based on many factors, such as weather conditions, clothing worn, intensity and duration of exercise, fitness level, age, menstrual cycle phase, and heat acclimation. This is why it is important to check it in different conditions and as you progress toward your triathlon goals.

You can search the Internet for instructions on how to do your own sweat rate testing—seeing how much you sweat under what conditions. Once you have collected some sweat rate data, you can start to fine-tune your fluid amounts. It's important to keep a detailed log as the tests require.

For example, if you sweat an average of 24 ounces (1 1/2 pounds) per hour on a seventy-degree day, then you can aim to drink 18 to 22 ounces per hour (75% to 90% of your losses in this example) in similar future conditions. No need to replace all hourly fluid losses—you want to be careful of overdrinking fluids (especially water!).

If you are a heavy *and* salty sweater, you can experiment with including more sodium in your fluids. Sodium is the primary electrolyte lost in sweat, so extra supplementation of this particular electrolyte during exercise has been shown to provide a variety of benefits. Not all sports drinks or electrolyte formulas are the same, so you may need to put on your sleuth hat to pick the better beverages. The marketing efforts put forth by beverage companies may lure you into thinking their product is the one and only—so read the labels.

Training Hydration Tips for the Every Woman Triathlete

- Everyone sweats different amounts in different training conditions and has her own tolerance level for dehydration. As a result, women's fluid needs vary, so see what works best for you.
- It is possible to overconsume fluids. To avoid drinking too much water during training, skip the gallon guzzle prior to and during workouts. On the other hand, too much sports drink can cause gastrointestinal distress, so start conservatively and adjust from there.

Training and Racing Nutrition

We could write an entirely separate book on training and racing nutrition. Furthermore, there are endless stories of nutrition goofs, records for who holds the most Porta-Potty stops, and DNFs (see page 235) due to poor (or nonexistent) nutrition strategies. Much detail is outside the scope of this book, but here are some highlights and pointers to get you going and finding your way.

First, a few definitions. *Training nutrition* encompasses nutrition before (pre-), during, and after your workout. *Racing nutrition* is similar, but this is your nutrition for your actual *race day*, no matter the distance or type of triathlon.

Training Nutrition

Keep a few considerations in mind as you start thinking about training nutrition. First, actually take the time to think about it. A common mistake among triathletes is to give utmost attention to triathlon training and yet forget that food actually can enhance (or ruin) performance. Even if you are just wanting to finish a race and you don't care about race times or the competitive aspect itself, you can still have a lousy race if you don't choose your nutrition wisely.

Remember to plan, try the plan, assess, and revise your nutrition plan. Rinse and repeat.

Preworkout nutrition can be relatively simple, but you need to bear in mind such factors as duration of the workout, intensity of the workout, time of day, and last meal eaten. Your preworkout nutrition can be a normal meal or snack you've eaten in the one to three hours prior, instead of added calories, especially if you are desiring weight loss. This is particularly the case if your workout is less than sixty to ninety minutes in duration.

As mentioned earlier, your body has in the range of 1,200 to 1,500 calories stored as carbohydrate. However, your body has *thousands more* calories stored as fat. By thousands, I mean over 80,000 calories for us Every Woman gals (as opposed to the Olympians!). This means, you can rely on your body to provide you with the fuel it is needs for these sixty- to ninety-minute (or less) workouts.

Preworkout nutrition should include a source of carbohydrate and a small amount of protein and/or fat. Examples include:

- Banana with peanut butter
- Cooked sweet potato with almond butter
- Yogurt with blueberries and chopped walnuts
- Oatmeal with pecans, strawberries, and milk of your choice
- Toast with mashed avocado
- Smoothie with milk of your choice, protein powder, fruit, and coconut oil

There really are endless combinations. You'll need to adjust the timing for when you eat and the amount for what you eat depending on the start time of your workout, in addition to honoring your hunger and any issues related to stomach or gut tolerance. This means your preworkout food could be consumed in the range of thirty minutes to two and a half hours in advance of your workout start time.

For your "during workout" nutrition, think about what workout you are doing (swim, bike, run, strength, or other cross-training), the duration, the intensity, and what you feel initially comfortable with. Remember, shorter workouts (60 to 90 minutes) simply do not require much nutrition—so keep it simple.

No need to try to add calories during a swim since you won't be able to easily eat during a race swim (and trust me, you won't want to). For the bike, consider your bike-handling skills and your comfort level in reaching for bike bottles (with liquid calories) versus reaching for food to eat while riding. For the run, there is the jostling of the stomach up and down as you run, along with a higher heart rate compared to the bike, so the same foods consumed on the bike may not go so well while running.

There are sports nutrition products aplenty on the market—bars, waffles, gels, blocks, gummies, beans, and powders. And then there are the many nonengineered food options, such as mini sandwiches, dried or fresh fruit, and homemade bars, bites, and gels. There's no "wrong" per se with what you choose except for when problems arise, such as gastrointestinal distress (identified by abdominal cramping, bloating, flatulence, diarrhea, vomiting). This can occur due to such factors as inadequate hydration, excessive calories, inappropriate source of calories (probably don't want to eat pizza!), or improper timing of calories. So, remember to find what works for you!

"Brick" and/or "mini tri" workouts are great to practice nutrition and fluid intake. This gives you a sense of what is working well (or not). Depending on when and what food and drink are consumed prior to the workout, you generally can aim for consuming 50 to 100 calories every thirty to sixty minutes. That's a big range—but remember, everyone is unique and you need to find what works for you.

For postworkout nutrition, think of this time period as an opportunity to keep your momentum going, as opposed to framing it with the classic reward-eating approach. Honestly, this is when a lot of athletes make decisions that nearly (or do) negate the workout they just completed. Instead of "Bring on *all* the food, ya'll; I earned this large pepperoni pizza and size-of-your-head Coke," it is preferable to switch to "Woo-hoo, I'm getting stronger and more fit! Let's keep this thang rollin' and eat quality food and keep kicking butt!" Traditional recommendations included pounding a sugar-laden protein drink (think chocolate milk) within thirty minutes to replenish. However, proper recovery nutrition is another "It depends" and not a black-or-white formula. We need to consider the type and duration of the workout you just completed (short vs. long, high intensity vs. aerobic-focused, strength vs. endurance, etc.), along with other factors, such as type of training block (for example, are you in a rest/recovery week or are you doing two training sessions a day?), weight-loss goals, protein and carbohydrate intake throughout the whole day, menstrual cycle phase, and so on. You can use "real food," instead of engineered sports nutrition products, as your postworkout nutrition and not force the thirty-minute window for shorter, aerobic-focused workouts, especially if you are eating optimal amounts of healthful items for the remainder of the day. A combination of quality protein (15 to 25 grams) and carbohydrate (20 to 60 grams) is ideal, which can easily be achieved with such foods as smoothies, "loaded" yogurts, and "smart" sandwiches or wraps.

If you are *not* postmenopausal, you may notice that some workouts seem more challenging in your high-hormone phase (generally, the few weeks prior to your period) or that you don't have as much oomph for higher-intensity workouts. If you experience this, give extra attention to your recovery nutrition and be sure to include quality sources of protein (no skimping!). You may need to shift up your overall calories, including those from carbohydrate, during this time of the month.

Racing Nutrition

In longer races, many triathletes like to load up on fuel on the bike, which is an okay strategy (albeit unnecessary many times) *if* you don't have gut issues when you run off the bike. In reality, your race day nutrition should be well practiced before race day arrives. So, race day is more the execution of what you have planned and practiced due to your excellent preparation! If things don't go the way you planned, then take notes for yourself after the race and brainstorm with someone who can help assess and fine-tune for the next go-round.

Training Nutrition Tips for the Every Woman Triathlete

- You'll hear nutrition tips from everyone, even Uncle Leon. While it's okay (and encouraged) to experiment, at least keep a journal for what seems to be working and what absolutely is not working. Be your own guide!
- In general, shorter and easier workouts do not require as much preworkout nutrition. Be careful of overloading your body in these circumstances.
- Nearly anything can work for your workout nutrition (yes, even pizza), but that doesn't mean it's the best for you or that it will make you go faster. Remember that your body has stored energy it can use and it can be taught to be more efficient with its energy sources depending on what you feed it. There's no need to go hawg wild!
- Always test your race day nutrition strategy at your anticipated race day effort one or more times prior to race day!
- Choose to "eat to nourish" instead of "eat to reward." See (and feel) how much better this is for your mind and body.

Now, go forth and fuel that awesome body of yours!

12 THE TRIFECTA: FAMILY, WORK, AND TRIATHLON

M OST OF THE TIME WHEN I TELL PEOPLE THAT I'M A WIFE AND a mother, they smile. Then, in the past, when I would say I'm a lawyer, I might see a mild grimace pass across their face. Finally, when I mention that I love triathlon (or worse, IRONMAN or long-distance racing), I see a horror-stricken expression, which is inevitably followed by, "What? How do you do it *all*? That's *craaaaazy*?"

You'll notice as you begin to balance your life, your family, your job, and your training, that surprisingly, you will feel *less* crazy. And the people around you will think you are *more* nuts. Also, you may tell others that you have a disorder—say, insomnia—to prevent them from feeling badly about the fact that you just accomplished more before six in the morning than they might in an entire day.

Balancing family and training is tough, I will not lie. To the point where I do not believe that balance is actually achievable at all. Something is always going to give—and henceforth you are required to juggle.

But your family can be a great strength to your training. I draw strength from my family during triathlon training and races. I also find my strength is *renewed*, and I am able to be a better wife, mother, and daughter after each training session. I may drop my kids off at the activity center, wanting to put them up for sale . . . but after a run, I pick them up and I am so glad to see them. The difference a few miles makes.

Admittedly, some families may be a detriment to your training. This is all part of the triathlon juggle. Where my family is a positive for me, my profession in the past was often the detriment. On the other hand, I have friends who work part-time or stay at home, but their families are completely unsupportive of their triathlon goals. We *all* must balance what we must balance. Once we balance, then we must balance some more. (Even though balance is sort of BS.)

In horse racing, a trifecta is a bet whereby the bettor must predict which horses will finish first, second, and third in that exact order. Family. Work. Triathlon. The Trifecta. Which horse is going to win? Does one horse have to win? Can you make them all win?

I receive e-mails all the time, saying the same things: *How do you do it all? I don't have time for it! I can't possibly find time to do a triathlon!* Well, yes, you *can*.

I often have my pompoms shaking and I'm screaming, "Yes, you can! Rah-rah! Shake your bon-bon! Ride your bike! Yah, yeah!" Because while "yes, you can be a triathlete" is very important, and is my big mantra, there is more to it. This Trifecta issue is also a question of your determination. The question is whether you are separating the "I can"s from the "I *won't*"s. The real question at the heart and start of this horse race is: *Do you have what it takes inside yourself to make your dreams happen? Or are you just a pile of empty, blubbering excuses?*

> nstead of saying, "How can I possibly get this done?" try saying, "I will get this done, and here's my plan for how to balance it all today."

This is your life, and it's up to you to make *your life* happen. Period. And it's up to you to make it happen without excuses, without finger pointing, without "can't"s and "but"s and "Well, I *would*, however . . ."

We women are always weighing the logistics of things: *How can I make this appointment between these hours? And who will pick up the kids? When can I find time to run? And forget swimming, who will do the laundry?*

At some point, we have to take responsibility for our health, our sanity, our jobs, and our families—and stop sacrificing ourselves for everyone else. Is life a sacrifice? Of course. But we need not be martyrs.

If you have put yourself in a position of martyrdom, lay down your shield. Time to rejuggle things. This is about you and your journey to yourself.

To make triathlon a part of your life, you must begin to look at your Trifecta differently. Instead of "How can I possibly get this done?" you need to say, "I will get this done, and here's my plan for how to juggle it all *today*."

Day by day, you make the plans. Not broad, sweeping, and unwavering plans. You may need to roll with the punches. The morning run might get rained out from a diaper explosion; *that's fine*; just get it done later *that* day. And if something tragic happens, then you move on and do better the next time. But you don't simply *allow yourself* an "out." You are better than that.

Women triathletes may feel guilty about putting ourselves first. We may be considered selfish and hardened by others, or maybe we think that of ourselves. Maybe we are scared that people will think we are lesser mothers and wives for leaving the family for a bike ride. Maybe we will get evil glances for showing up with wet hair at a family reunion or PTA meetings.

But I say it all the time: what good are we to others when we feel like crap about ourselves? Do not worry about what others think about you. Take care of yourself. Make time. Prioritize and plan, and your Trifecta will be three beautiful, manageable horses.

DOING IT ALL

A few months into my structured triathlon training, I found myself completely frustrated at home and at work. I woke up at 4:30 a.m., completed everything I was supposed to do that day, including training, plus feeding/entertaining/getting beat up by children after my workday was over. By the end of the day, I was at the end of my rope, sick of doing everything for everyone. I was deadly sick of the practice of law. I was also incredibly sore from the training that morning . . . but interestingly, the sore muscles were the best part of *that particular* day.

I realized something fairly early in the triathlon game. Sometimes when I felt as though I was losing my mind at home or at work, the promise of triathlon and training *saved* me. The promise of the next workout and the quiet and the sweat began to be a foundation of sanity for me.

I could murder the Expert right now, but at least I have a seven-mile run to think of the many reasons that I shouldn't. Coincidentally, by the time I was finished with 7 miles, I was thinking of all the ways I loved the man and looked forward to seeing him at dinner.

Did that butthead partner actually ask me, "Did you really go to law school?" I'll slash the tires on his midlife crisis car! I'll toss his Rolex in the river! A few thousand meters later, I was armed with the power to continue briefing and smiling (most of the time).

Triathlon is an enigma: how can something *so* painful also be relaxing and therapeutic? How can a sport save you from jail time?

I slowly began to understand the complexity of the triathlon balance and how it was actually saving my life. Saving. My. Life. When every single other thing in my life was making me bat-shit crazy, triathlon was keeping me balanced and sane. On challenging days, triathlon was sometimes the only thing that I could snuggle to and feel safe. *I love you, swim cap. You are the world to me, running shoes. Thank you for loving me, bicycle.*

Of course, triathlon is not my *life*. But it is an important part of my life. Swimming, biking, and running made clear the blessings around me. Triathlon became the *process* that allowed me to see my life for all its good, all the things worth loving and living for.

Triathlon is all about learning to prioritize. I do not think training for an IRONMAN is too much to ask out of my life. However, I am strongly convinced that cleaning my house is waaaaaay too difficult to squeeze into my schedule. Therefore, the swim workout usually wins. And cleaning the house loses. My health and training takes priority over a white-glove-clean house . . . sorry, but it's true. (Very, very true.)

MARRIAGE AND SERIOUS RELATIONSHIPS

Marriage is one of life's greatest joys —and one of its most enormous pains. Marriage combined with triathlon is like a giant Slurpee—delicious and beautiful—but most often causing an enormous headache and horrors to your waistline. The same can be said for long-term relationships. Anytime you are cooped up and sharing bathrooms with someone you *love*, you will have issues.

There are three possible scenarios where you are the triathlete in your marriage or serious relationship:

1. You are the solo triathlete and your significant other is *supportive*.
2. You are the solo triathlete and your significant other is *not supportive* or is *indifferent*.
3. You are both triathletes.

No matter which category you fall into, it is *all* a personal battle and one that you must fight smartly and strategically.

The Solo Triathlete, Supportive Partner

I have a longtime girlfriend who is a stay-at-home mom. Her husband works full-time, but when he walks in the door, she takes off for training. On weekends? She's gone riding and bricking and swimming. The dude drags the kids to the races to watch her race. He's totally cool with it. He makes posters. He cheers. He is a rarity and she's quite lucky to have this kind of undying support.

If you are in a comparable situation, I think the danger is taking the saintly significant other for granted. Eventually, I would imagine he might tire of your being gone every available moment to spend time with your bike. So, be grateful for what you have, but be careful not to take advantage or create a resentment that is unnecessary in your pretty-darn-perfect training world. And you should probably do some nice things for that partner of yours, too—and I don't mean cooking (although that is a nice start).

The Non-supportive Butthead Partner

You are living with a non-supportive butthead. You're darn right that I don't know you and I *just* called your partner a butthead. This situation is *the worst*. You have a new passion (triathlon) that will benefit your life. But your significant other is negative, unsupportive, or abusive (or all three).

These situations call for you to be a triathlon ninja. If you are not a ninja, you will never make it to your first (or next) race. Do not attempt to stick the butthead with the kids while you go on a bike ride. Do not even bother explaining to the butthead that you can't [insert whatever chore it is] because you have a long run. You will be setting a time bomb.

Without delving into the issues that may be at the root of your relationship—and assuming you want to stay in the relationship, you *must* bend over backward to ensure that the other person is *in no way* inconvenienced by your triathlon dreams. You must complete workouts before the butthead is awake. Learn to love your slow cooker and cook every darn meal in it. Find other childcare for your race days. You must never leave the butthead with screaming kids or dirty laundry while you go for a run. Sell your stuff on eBay to pay for your new triathlon suit. Don't even leave room for them to say, "How much did *that* cost *me*?" (And don't sell *their* stuff!)

Is this really fair? *Heck no, Joe!* But do you want to be a triathlete and still stay in the relationship, or what?

Remember that you cannot change the actions of others. You can only change yourself and how you react to their actions. Get up really early. Squeeze in the workouts. Find ways to make quick meals, have laundry delivered to your office, or whatever it takes. Make it happen and talk about your training with others who *will* be supportive.

You must find a way for your butthead partner to have absolutely no ammunition against you. That said, here's a very serious note: if you are in an abusive situation, then you should seek help and get out immediately. Find someone in your triathlon group, tell her you are being abused, and move in with her. Then, you can bike and train to your heart's content. In all seriousness, seek help.

Finally, do not bother to tell your good triathlon stories to your partner if he or she will do nothing but rain on your parade. Find something else to talk about together (such as why your significant other is such a butthead . . . okay, not that).

The best you can hope is that your butthead partner will begin to see the changes in your life and warm up to the new you. Maybe even come along for the ride. We can hope for that. If the butthead *does* join you, then you must implement a new policy going forward, requiring that your partner be nice and supportive if he or she wants to come along and play with the cool people. And if he or she declines? That's okay. It may take time to turn your partner into a triathlete as well.

The Two-Athlete Compromise

When you have two people training for triathlon, be prepared for some of the strangest fights: *No, I get to swim first! Me! I'm first! Did you take the last water bottle? How could you be so inconsiderate?! What? You lost my IRONMAN visor?! Get off my bicycle! Those are my gels! You are not getting a new helmet—I need one first!*

You must compromise often, and negotiate as if in a constant hostage situation. A two-triathlete household is tough. Is it tougher than being married to someone who is *not* into triathlon? Who knows. But if you are asking your significant other to watch kids for hours on end or spend time alone much of the weekend, or take on the responsibilities of the house while you are out on your bike, you are either (1) married to a saint (see the first scenario, above); or (2) cooking a recipe for disaster (see the second scenario).

For me, I would have been just fine doing triathlon alone, without the Expert. But I am also no fool in my house. I knew that the man would *never* agree to let me vanish for five-hour bike rides and two-hour runs on a weekend, saying, *Have fun with the kids, sucker!* He's (admittedly) just not that kind of character.

The *only* way to live in harmony in my house with triathlon *and* the Expert . . . was to pull him into the sport with me. So, I signed *him* up for races. He trained, we found babysitters, and he's a triathlete now, too. It's not that the Expert would have been unsupportive of my triathlon dreams . . . it's just that he doesn't want to be stuck solo with the kids for seven hours while I'm out having a good ole time. And I can't say that I blame him.

Now for a word about partners in general. *Sigh*.

The Expert came along without much convincing. Some partners may require more convincing (not nagging). However, others may come along just because *they* have something to prove. If their significant other is out there kicking triathlon butt, and *they* are sitting on *their* butt—eventually, their ego might not be able to take it—and they will come running just to *prove* that they can beat their partner at her own game (whether it's true or not).

That may be one way to get partners involved—pure and simple peer pressure. If they do come along and they are having a coronary the first time they run—go easy, let them "enjoy" the sport and focus on a team effort to bring them into triathlon. The long-run benefits for the family or relationship just might be magical.

As far as scheduling in the two-triathlete house, the Expert and I have found that making a simple training compromise calendar and sticking it on the refrigerator alleviates *some* of the arguments surrounding workout times. On my early-morning workouts, the Expert is home with the kids or we have a sitter come in early so we can both go work out. On his early-morning workouts, I am home with the kids.

When you get into long-distance training, sometimes the calendar is the only thing that makes sense, and prevents arguments and hurt feelings.

Our workout calendar has looked something like this:

Day of Week	Me	The Expert
*Sunday	Long ride/run	Morning workout (gym with kids)
Monday	Recovery	Morning workout
Tuesday	Morning workout (Babysitter in early so both can train early)	Morning workout
Wednesday	Morning workout	Evening workout
Thursday	Evening workout	Morning workout
Friday	Morning workout	Recovery
*Saturday	Morning workout (gym with kids)	Long ride/run

Marriage Ain't Easy

To say that our marriage was delightful over the past almost-decade would be a dirty rotten lie. We had a solid marriage for quite a few years, but throwing kids into the mix was insane for us. Thus, we have struggled, even to the point of discussing the big "D" word.

Several times. *Divorce. Divorce. Ugh.*

We always decide against it, which is sometimes because of love, sometimes because of history, sometimes because of the kids. And sometimes because of sheer laziness and not wanting to divide up our things. "It's *my* couch."

Triathlon initially tore us apart, but then brought us closer back together (and arguably once again farther apart during IRONMAN, and then back together again). It was hard to get rolling together with the training because we had been so lazy, so stressed for many years. The Expert resented me for holding him back from his cycling and running in the early days of our marriage. I felt terrible for the way I had acted back then, but I had profusely apologized and was trying to move forward. He, understandably, wanted to punish me for it. So, training *almost* felt like another hurdle to overcome.

But overcome it, we did. And overcome it, we continue to do—perhaps that's marriage and has nothing to do with triathlon. Perhaps.

Even now, sometimes the Expert will see me come in from a long workout and say, disbelieving, "Who *are* you and what have you done with my wife?" Only now, he means it in a good way.

One of the hardest parts about marriage, friendships, and all relationships is when one person changes. The other person is often left standing there, thinking, *What just happened to my person?* Whether it's changing for the "good" or the not-so-great, change is hard. Learning to accept changes in ourselves might seem easy—but the other people, who are accustomed to us being certain ways—we must give them a second to breathe. It's easy to say, "Take me as I am now or else!" but that's neither productive nor well-received.

Date on a Workout

Sunday long rides became a thing for the Expert and me leading up to our first IRONMAN 70.3. We easily rode 40 to 50 miles on a given weekend morning. We had a babysitter come in for the weekend rides and while we arguably spent a small fortune on early-morning childcare during this time, we considered it money we would have otherwise spent going out to dinner and drinks in our former, non-triathlon-addicted life. We simply shifted the finances elsewhere.

Our summer bike routine was easy:

Early rise around 5:30 a.m.

Get in some sort of fight because we were tired or because one of us (the Expert) was not moving quickly enough for the Schedule Tyrant (me);

After fussing at him and him telling me to jump off a bridge, the angry Expert would load up the car; and

I'd stomp around the house equally mad, but trying not to wake the children.

The night before the ride, we'd warn the children as to which babysitter they would wake up to. The kids were resilient. After we had been training for a few months, James would ask me, "Who is coming tomorrow to play with us?"

"Oh, nobody, baby. Daddy and I rode yesterday. It's Mommy and Daddy today," I would say.

"Aw, man," James said. "I don't want to play with you, Mommy."

"Well, you got Mom today," I said.

Stella would then chime in against me, "You ride your bike, Mommy."

"Yes," James said. "Go ride your bike."

Needless to say, the kids enjoyed having some young person to run them ragged for a few hours while the Expert and I killed ourselves on the bikes.

You can learn to date differently. It's possible.

PARENTHOOD

I thought the movie *Parenthood* was just a comedy. Actually, certain parts of that movie were filmed at our house. (Who knew?!) Children are absolutely a blessing—and children will make you absolutely insane— all at once.

Triathlon allows me a much-needed escape, and gives me *permission* to take care of myself. Triathlon has made me a better, more patient mother, and has brought my young children into the fold of swim, bike, run, and fitness . . . which is incredibly exciting.

Setting the Example

You may feel guilty taking time away from your kids for triathlon. But I urge you to put it in perspective. You are teaching the children wonderful lessons about health and perseverance. Stay the course.

After nearly ten years in the sport, I can affirmatively say that being a tri mom has only positively influenced my children. My kids see healthy mom. My kids run and move because I do, because my husband does. They are used to seeing healthy food; they know what it is.

Part of the reason I do triathlon, part of the reason I spend weekends running, and most important, the reason I am *capable* of telling my kids good-bye to go for a swim, is simple. I want my children to see the motion, to understand the weirdness (beauty) of waking up at unholy hours to run, bike, and swim. Then, I want them to think it's no big deal to do so. (Oh, and I need some stinking time to myself!)

I look back and realize that their little unit was awesome. I want my kids to be healthy and to crave competition and movement. I hope they find a bike ride to be fun, not work. I hope they want to run with their nerdy parents.

The Expert and I love to watch videos of the past years' IRONMAN World Championship. Sometimes the kids will watch with us. One night, Stella saw Mirinda Carfrae, the 2010 IRONMAN World Champion, and screamed, "Ohhhh, there's Mommy!"

And then James said, "No, it's not. That's Daddy!"

Of course, neither I nor the Expert was in Kona in 2010 (vacation, racing, or otherwise).

Then, Stella hopped off my lap and took off running. She ran loops around the house, screaming, "I running! I like Mommy! I runnnnnning!"

James chimed in: "No, I am running like Mommy, too!"

They continued running and arguing about who was running faster. Even though the Atwood House Rules disallow running inside the house, I let them go. In that moment, I felt it. I knew that I was doing right by my children, by my triathlon example, however small it was. In that space, I felt that my two babies would run and play and have their sweaty lives right out in front of them. They would be healthy and happy. And run. And sweat. And *love* it. Even if they choose not to race, then at least, the rug rats will know that it was a possibility. The Swim Bike Kids are older now, and they love sports and doing active things. They have done some triathlons, and the option to become a triathlete for both of them is wide open. But they get to decide, and just knowing that they *can* be triathletes—if they simply decide to? That's priceless.

Think about those things as you embark on your journey. Yes, it will be hard to leave and not see your kids sometimes in the mornings. You may miss them at night because you are running or swimming. But I promise you, they will benefit a million times more from a healthy, happy mother who misses some frosted cereal mornings—than an unhealthy, sad mom who was just around all the time.

Single Moms

If you are a single mother, then you've got a whole other set of challenges in the world of triathlon. But hopefully, you can find ways to compromise with your saintly babysitters and find time to train. You *especially*—don't feel bad being away from your kids! You are their mom—*and* dad and grandparents sometimes, too. So, you *definitely* need a break. You are teaching them good things by your healthy example. Remember: it's not unfair to have time to yourself. You are bringing yourself back as a better mother and human being: a supermom.

Finding Your Quiet

I grew up an only child, so my surroundings were pretty quiet. I am wired to appreciate the solitary time, the stillness.

Well. Years and years later, I became a parent. I had no earthly idea how loud parenting would be. My parents did not warn me. Parenting *me* had been pretty quiet for them, also.

But the two kids that sprang forth from my—well, you know—they are *insanely* loud. To be frank and to the horror of helicopter parents everywhere, I love triathlon mostly because it gives me a break away from my loud house and active munchkins. Sometimes the whiny kids, the horrible sounds of that blasted *Caillou* boy on the television and the breaking of my lamps and tables bothers me *so* much that I would rather suffer on a bike *for hours on end* than be at home with the circus monkeys.

Am I selfish? Maybe.

But really, I think I'm admitting that I am human. I am admitting that I have a breaking point. And that breaking point happens to be my lamps. Do I love my kids? Of course, more than anything. Do I *like* my kids? Yes, about 68 percent of the time. But when I have time off to swim and bike and run, I come back feeling like a real human again . . . and the *like* number goes up to around 93 percent. See, it's really simple math.

Mom x (Swim + Bike + Run) = Mommy is nice
See? Very basic math.

The *Mom*-Crunched Triathlete

I have a magnet on my fridge that says: "What Would You Do, If You Knew You Could Not Fail?" I love this question, because my answer never changes. If I could not fail, I would be a writer, an athlete, and a good wife and mother. Three (four?) things I want more than anything in this world, and the things I strive for on a daily basis.

Chris Carmichael wrote *Time-Crunched Triathlete* book.[1] *Time-crunched* is an understatement for most women. But it begs the question: are you *mom*-crunched (the nirvana state of time-crunched, haggard, and exhausted)? Is your time *so* crunched that you can't see straight? And if so . . . how do you survive it, let alone take on triathlon? Perhaps a better question is: how do your children survive? (I guess we can worry about them later.)

Here's my best advice for when the motherhood plane is going down—put on *your* oxygen mask first, and then:

Be Mom and Be Awesome

Yes, you can be *both* a mom and awesome. You can be a mom and a triathlete/runner/cyclist/chess champion (insert whatever you think is awesome here). You should go after what you think is awesome. Remember that *you* were here first. Take care of you. If you fail to take care of yourself, you are a useless pet rock to those around you. Stop wishing and start doing! Once you begin to *do*, do not feel guilty about the time you spend *doing*.

Remind yourself that you are ingraining healthy ideals into your family: when they see you fall down on your bike and get back up, you are demonstrating a few lessons. The first lesson is to get back up when you fall. The second lesson is: never pay attention to Mommy when it comes to bike-handling skills.

Nod and Smile

When the nonbusy, nonimportant people of your world request stupid things of you that take you away from your family, work, or training, remember to simply nod and smile, knowing that you have no intention of doing anything they ask.

By the nod and smile, the asker will find you polite. Then, when you simply "forget" to bake that sunshine pie for the non-triathlon-related fund-raiser, you can pretend to be horrifically embarrassed, wave your hands and blame it on your impossibly busy life. (Note: From experience, I know that you can pull off the nod and smile *only twice per social function/group*. On the third time, you must say yes and deliver. And by "deliver," I mean go to Safeway and buy that "homemade" pie.)

Pee and Move

This is an important lesson in triathlon and in life. You need to *go* where you can and get a move on. You think your bathroom time is your quiet time? Then, you must have some seriously polite children. There's no time for potty in racing! Go, go, go! Either way, there is a time to learn to get it done and move on.

Take Care of Your Toes

Triathletes and runners are prone to contract the dreaded black toenail, calluses, and other nasty foot things. Just remember to paint your toenails every once in a while. The little splash of color will make you feel human. I promise. Even when you come in from a run and your toddler wipes a booger right on your big toe and screams, "So pretty, Mommy!"

You just smile and say, "You're darn right, kid. Those are manicured toes. Take notice!"

Sleep. Run. Do the Nasty. Repeat.

Just do *it*. Yes, *it*. You'll feel better. And whoever's on the receiving end might make you breakfast and say nice things about you the next day.

Whatever.

So, just do it because you'll feel better. Endorphins.

Ask for Help

Find some good friends, neighbors, or teenagers who will watch your offspring while you go on a long run or ride.

If you are riding solo or if your other half is not a triathlete, as discussed earlier, he or she will need a break, too. Get a sitter so the other half can see the latest sci-fi movie while you are out playing fancy Orca in your wetsuit. Who knows, this special consideration might lead to a little more of the "nasty" from the previous step.

Asking for help can also be from strangers for such chores as grocery delivery or house-cleaning. It's worth it.

Eat Well

Historically, I would not be the one to talk about nutrition or diet or anything other than peanut butter and the deliciousness of all things Dairy Queen. But over time, I have learned that nutrition is so important and no, not just about weight loss or dieting. You read about nutrition earlier, so maybe you're thinking, *Yeah, yeah, Meredith, I get it.* Nutrition is important to your performance in life, your mood, the way you feel about yourself, the colds you get (or don't). I have personally correlated the food I put in my face to the feelings and words that come out of my mouth. I am nicer, kinder, and san(er) when I eat well.

Put Yourself in Timeout

Overtraining, overworked, overstressed? If you don't put yourself in a timeout, then God might put you in timeout, and you may not like what he decides. God once broke my foot to make me slow down and appreciate my life. *I kid you not*. God later gave me a stress fracture and also tendinitis. For those of you in the Bible Belt screaming that God is not a vengeful God, yes, okay. But he likes to slow me down when I get out of control by giving me things that *will* get my attention.

When are you losing your mind from work, life, and training, just take a rest day—haul out your crayons and coloring books and doodle. Whatever floats your sanity boat. It is a tough job being a hero. Sometimes you need to prop up your feet, be lazy with the kids, and give those red, knee-high Wonder Woman boots a day off.

Make It Happen

Remember Gerry's wisdom: "You have a duty to *yourself* to find a way to get things done—rather than finding an excuse for why you didn't."

So, you gotta figure it out. Make time for your children, make time for training, and handle your business at work/home/wherever you are beckoned. Something inevitably "gives" when a new project is added.

You must pull it all together and make it look pretty, functional, and awesome. (Hopefully, no one will pull back the curtain and see the She Wizard—with all the Scotch tape and stretch marks.)

Remember Your People

The kiddos were around the ages of four and five during the year I tackled my first IRONMAN. Now, I don't recommend trying to do the insanity that is IRONMAN training with a four- and a five-year-old, a full-time job, and all the responsibilities that come with life and being a parent. But, once I committed to the dream I was into it, and the family was thrown onto the roller coaster with me.

(Hindsight really *is* 20/20.)

Looking back, I can see that while I balanced the kid responsibilities and family fun (reasonably, sometimes) well, many other things seriously fell off the radar. My marriage struggled big time—we almost called it quits that year. All in all, I would say that the road to that big IRONMAN dream was paved with tacks, oil, and lots of wounds—training injuries, financial difficulties, and emotional scars to boot.

I dragged my family with me straight to my dream—without ever bothering to ask them how they felt about it all.

"It's *my* dream, after all." *Ack*.

The culmination of *my* big year was at the finish line of IRONMAN Coeur d'Alene. My family (parents, the Expert, and my sweet girl and sweet boy) made the big trip. The cannon went off at swim start, and my family began the long day of sit, wait, and cheer for one of the slowest and least accomplished racers out there on the course.

We had planned everything well, so that the family could go back to the rental house and rest, sleep, and hang out while I was climbing the mountains. But still, long-distance racing can be a really long day for spectators—no matter how much they love you.

On my first loop of the run, around Mile 6, I saw my dad against the fence—and I hugged him. I looked over to the trees to see my mom with one kiddo asleep in her lap and another kiddo stuffing cookies into his face. He waved, I waved. My heart was so full. *These people love me enough to stand out here for literally hours to watch this ridiculousness. How blessed am I?*

At the Mile 13 turnaround, the Expert informed me that I had to hustle to be sure to make the cutoff, and I was like, "I am hustling, dude. This *is* my hustle."

But I listened, made note of the pace I had to keep, and I went. I was going to cross the finish line about sixteen minutes before the seventeen-hour cutoff time—I had done it. I turned onto the last street and ran and smiled and cried the seven blocks into the finish chute, hearing those words, "You are an IRONMAN."

The lights were blinding. And the dream was captured. *Yesssssss!*

A few minutes after the medal was placed around my neck, I found my family.

My dad looked as though he had been through a war zone.

My mom was crying—happy tears, but she looked so worn.

The Expert was smiling, but looked beaten.

My daughter was in full kid-tantrum mode.

Lastly, my intuitive and sensitive five-year-old James was crying and clinging to me as if it was the end of days.

Apparently, he had waited all day long for something. He had been told *all day long* by the Expert that I would high-five him at the finish.

Great, right? I could have high-fived my kid. Easy!

However, I didn't know that was the actual plan. I didn't think about it, as I had seen them a few times—leaving transition, I had kissed them all. I had seen my daughter at Mile 13, and hugged her.

But I missed the memo to stop, look, and listen in the finish chute. The issue, though, is that I *should* have thought to stop. But through the blinding lights and the emotion, I just *didn't*. I didn't stop to look for my family.

Again, hindsight is so clear. Of course, now, I would stop and search and look for them. But this was *my* first IRONMAN. *Me. Me. Mine. Mine. Me.*

To this day, the thought of missing my son's high five is a recurring nightmare for me.

I sometimes think about it, and I literally weep about it. I do actually dream about it. *How could I have been so selfish and stupid?* The culmination of events leading up to that race was massive, and the crew was all right there with me. Sometimes fighting me, sometimes accepting me—but *always with me*.

And leave it up to me to muck it up in the end. I had swung for the wall and hit the proverbial home run—and yet I had struck out completely.

Because with that first IRONMAN, I had caused a ripple, a wake, and a wave of sadness, mess, and minor scars that I can see *now*.

The situation isn't helped by the fact that my son, now eleven, is the kid with the elephant memory: "Mom, remember that race in the dark when I was five and you forgot to high-five me?" (Super.) Never mind that the next race, only twelve weeks later, I carried treats and stopped and hugged and high-fived no less than *twelve* times, including a massive finish chute victory hug and dance.

My too-little, too-late efforts didn't matter. *That* is not what is remembered. Forgetting my sweet family, my sweet boy, in *my* important moment is what *he* remembers.

Now, years and years later, when I think about IRONMAN Coeur d'Alene, that's what I remember, too. I remember my first IRONMAN as a time when I found myself and rose up against the odds to complete one of the most difficult courses in America.

Then, I deeply remember it as a moment where I forgot the most important people in my life, for a span of months, and then really drove it home in the eleventh hour.

And that memory completely overshadows the glory for me.

Each race since Coeur d'Alene has been different. I crossed the line of Beach2Battleship with both of our kids in 2014, which my daughter thought rocked to no end. She was thrilled. My son? Not so much.

He still mentions the *other* one—the one in the dark where I forgot.

Right now, I would trade in all my finishes—every last one of them— to go back and fix that moment. And of course, I can't. But I can remember with every workout and every day, that triathlon is not *my* everything. It's *a lot* and it is a big part of me, but it is not *me*.

Triathlon is not *who* I am: I am a wife, a mom, a daughter, a granddaughter, a friend, a writer, an entrepreneur, a silly person who loves peanut butter. I am all of those things first—before a triathlete, and long before an IRONMAN. I will not forget who is important. I will not forget what matters. I will *always* look for my family or friends in the finish chute of these grueling, all-day races—and going forward, I may stand there, like a statue until I find them. Sure, I may miss a PR, but I will never (ever) again miss the moment of joy that is so deservedly *theirs* to share.

I tell this story in this book about first triathlons, because I want each and Every Woman to read my experience and *know* better—from the outset. That triathlon, while I truly believed it saved me—has turned out not to *be* me. Maybe you would know to high-five, regardless. But just in case, now you can't unknow. Go forth and find your people in the crowd.

WORK

Triathlon made me more alert and thus, a better employee. Even though most days, I wanted to swim, bike, and run my way right out of the legal profession. Eventually, I guess I did. Some people are born lawyers. I am not one of them.

Many (many) jobs can be quite soul-sucking. During the beginning of my triathlon expedition, I was having trouble sleeping from all the work I had to do. Those whispering files sitting on my desk, the list of to-dos, the things I should be drafting, reading, reviewing. More endless lists of statutes, opinions, and cases I would never find time to read. So, so many lists.

Triathlon became a big bonus to my endless lists. When I plopped my head on the pillow each night, I found myself worrying about my morning workout instead of the whispering files at the office. I was forced to barrel through the workout *before* I could get to the files. In a strange way, triathlon put up a manageable *barrier* to my job. I would deal with the job when I finished doing something for myself.

And while the files were still there, churning in my head, I could only see them in abstract. I could not reach them or hear them or do anything while I was underwater or out on the bike. The sights and sounds of triathlon drowned out the job when I most needed it drowned out.

I liked that.

The Working Mom Dilemma

Whether you work full-time, part-time, from home or as a stay-at-home wife and mother, your time is precious and tough to find. I swear (and I will swear this until kingdom come), that the best bet to make this triathlon thing work is to accomplish your training first thing in the morning.

But I'm not a morning person, you whine. Suck it up, buttercup! Races are in the morning. Babies cry and wake up in the morning. *Good Morning America* or the *Today Show* is on the television in the morning. Those people are awake! You can do it.

The bonus about the morning workouts? First, usually the house is quiet and the rest of the world is asleep. This is a good time to get your thoughts together, make your mental lists, and find some motivational quiet time.

Additionally, you are less likely to skip the workout if you knock it out first thing. I find it virtually impossible to accomplish a 6:30 p.m. workout after a hard day at work. Something always comes up and blows my nighttime workout. Or I am too tired. I just do not like it. For me, morning is rarely disturbed. Also, the morning workout makes me have a better day at work. I am more focused, energized, and I feel better having done something for myself before working for the Dude.

As I mentioned earlier, if you find a gym near where you work, the morning workouts may be even better. Or sometimes, you can squeeze in a lunchtime run. Of course, when and where you work out is going to depend on your life, your circumstances. If evening is better for you, heck, if 11 p.m. is better for you, rock out. Remember, it is up to *you* to make it happen.

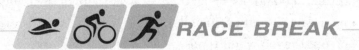 RACE BREAK

Paratriathlon and Tri-ing with Disability

When I began tri-ing, I would often complain about my feet hurting me. I would whine about my knees, my hips, and my ankles giving me trouble. Then, I began to learn a little about paratriathlon, the heroic athletes and individuals who are training for triathlon in the midst of physical disabilities, such as paralysis and limb loss.

continues

continued

If you complain about your fatness or your aching knees, there is nothing like a visit with a paratriathlete to bring you back down to earth. One of the most important times in my life happened during a lunch with my friend Mike Lenhart. One of his athletes, Kelly Casabere, joined us for lunch. Kelly is a single amputee who lost her left leg above the knee after a boating accident in high school. She competed in her first triathlon only a year prior and she also plays soccer. She smiled and laughed, her joy was infectious. I wanted to ask Kelly how she wasn't angry or sad about her limb loss. I really could not bear to ask such a negative question in such a positive presence. But selfishly, I had to know. So, I asked her anyway.

She said, "There is no reason to be angry when I stared death in the face. And I won. Every day is a gift."

Where There's a Wheel

During my time as a triathlete, I have met amazing, inspirational individuals with disabilities who have proven truly that anything is possible.

From Scott Rigsby (double-amputee finisher at Kona) to the Pease brothers—Kyle and Brent—who compete in IRONMAN, I have learned that heart, soul, and community are the legs and bodies that allow us to cross the finish lines. If you need some inspiration or want to get involved, check out such amazing organizations as the Scott Rigsby Foundation (scottrigsbyfoundation.org) and the Kyle Pease Foundation (kylepeasefoundation.org). Within these communities, if you are an able-bodied athlete, you will learn what an amazing gift your able body is. If you are not so able-bodied, then you will find an instant community filled with others who have limitations and disabilities but make the best of their gifts to move forward and across finish lines.

13 TRI THROUGH TOUGH TIMES

I N January 2012, I had an Ironman 70.3 under my belt. However, I was struggling to be grateful and proud of myself. I tried to remind myself how far I had come in just a little over a year. But something wasn't resonating. I felt, well, just let down.

The Expert and I headed out for a 45-mile bike ride, trying to get geared up for the *second* 70.3 race coming up in April. At Mile 32, I dismounted my bike and waited until the Expert rolled back to me. I was hurting and tired and angry. I looked at the Expert and said, "I'm not doing this anymore."

He stared at me. "You have to. You have, like, thirteen miles to get home."

"No. I mean I don't want to do *this* anymore. This training. Triathlon. This this *this*!" I said, flailing my arms.

I'm not sure what caused it. Yes, I was tired from a recent trip. Yes, the ride was the longest one in a while. Yes, my second 70.3 was creeping scary close.

But the quitting *feeling* was something bigger.

The temperature was forty degrees. My hands and feet were completely frozen from the ride. My kids were at home with a babysitter. It was a Sunday afternoon. It was a perfectly good day, and I was *suffering* on a bike, when I could have been hanging out with my kids, reading Elmo, shopping or watching a movie or organizing a closet. But instead, I was physically hurting myself, freezing my tail off, and doing it all *on purpose*. At Mile 32, I just couldn't take it anymore.

The Expert continued riding. He knows when I slip into crazy, to move along. He had his phone and said to call if I had a mechanical problem.

I rode a few miles, stopped, and sat on a bench. I did this a few times. I was hungry. I was tired, so tired of it all. *How did I go from motivated to falling flat out of space?*

I wasn't able to pep myself up, talk myself out of it, put my "Yes, you can" motivation tactic to work on myself. I just gave up for no real reason. The following day started out no better.

I woke up to complete chaos. Our daughter was sick. After taking her to the doctor, I dragged myself into the gym, missing the entire morning of work. I had also missed the scheduled indoor cycling class. So, it was just me, sitting in the dark cycling studio on a Spin bike . . . by myself.

I sat on the front row under the dim lights and turned on Snow Patrol (instead of something peppier). I held on for the misery. I stared at myself in the mirror for the first fifteen minutes while I rode. Just bore a hole through my image with my beady, crabby little sad eyes. I stared and stared. Until, little by little, my legs picked up speed. Then, my heart rate climbed. The sweat started pouring off my visor. Thirty minutes later, I was pushing my heart rate into Zone 4.

An hour later, I was back on the triathlon high. In fact, I felt so good that I skipped on over to the treadmill and ran 2 miles for fun. Then, I drove home.

The memory of the terrible ride from the day before was gone. And just like that, my head was back in the triathlon game. (Part of my new good mood *may* have been missing work that morning, but we'll leave that out of the equation for now.)

The simple answer to all of these "I quit" emotions is simple: *Just keep moving forward*. I will repeat this until I am blue in the face. If the day is bad, you must just close up shop and focus on the next day. Because the next day just might turn out fantastic. Don't give up.

EVERYONE IS STRUGGLING

I am a big fan of the business magazine *Inc*. In the November 2011 issue, I found an amazing one-page article titled "Stop Feeling Like a Big Fat Loser." Well, *that* got my attention. I read on:

> "If nobody shares they are struggling, nobody will know anybody else is struggling. That results in a bunch of people feeling isolated and scared and like big, fat losers."[1]

I find this so true in everyday life. Some people are intensely private and shuffle along in life preferring to have others glean nothing personal about them, see no faults, smell no farts, and only observe them flying high in their externally perfect world. I also understand that people may be introverts and that sharing goes against their very nature. (I am not criticizing being an introvert.) People e-mail me often: "OMG, I can't believe you wrote that!"

> "The hardest thing in life is knowing which bridge to cross, and which bridge to burn."
>
> —DAVID RUSSELL

This was especially true after I shared all the food I ate after my half IRONMAN 70.3 race, my wetsuit experiences, and the millions of posts on my size. I have never lied about how hard it is to be a mother, especially a working mother. How sometimes marriage sucks. I figured that I was doing no good to anyone by candy-coating my journey. Most of all, I would be no good to myself.

Everyone struggles in life, in triathlon. The more I wrote over the years, the more I began to understand the importance of sharing struggles, adventures, and advice with others.

In the triathlon context, I encourage advanced members of the sport to recall where they started and to always maintain a spirit of *encouragement* to baby triathletes—even slow or unfit babies. I remember people who said/say encouraging things to me; I remember those who didn't/don't. Words matter big time to the "little" people wearing swim caps and spandex for the first time. I find, for the most part, triathletes are some of the most amazing, encouraging, and supporting group of athletes. But every bunch of bananas has their monkeys . . . so . . .

On your journey, remember to share your experiences more often. Even if you are an introvert—you can certainly find one person at your gym to encourage—and that makes a difference. One of my most encouraging triathlete friends, Karen (who I call "Yoda" because she is so wise), is a pretty quiet person—but she *quietly* offers me wise, balanced, and genius advice. She shares her triathlon knowledge freely and has helped me more than she knows. Yoda pays it forward. *Share you must.*

If you can bravely stomach sharing your fears and struggles in an open forum, such as a blog or a seminar (or a book?!), I encourage you to do it! Chances are, if you are feeling low or "like a big fat loser," someone else is feeling the same way. If we can all help one another become better people and stronger triathletes, we should do it. Really, what is the point of faking it? Everyone knows faking it is just for the bedroom and cocktail parties.

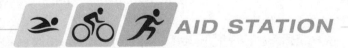 **AID STATION**

DOING THE BEST WE CAN

One of my favorite gratitude moments happened on a day I was scheduled to run 11 miles, which would be a new milestone. I was scared. I had run barely 10 miles the week before.

The morning was hot and quiet. I ran out 5.5 miles without issue. Then, I made the turnaround and a little while later, I saw two big guys running toward me. I was alarmed for a minute, but then I realized they

continues

continued

were jogging. Two men who appeared to be a father and son, running directly toward me. I'll call them Fred and Ben. Fred is the dad in this story.

The most remarkable thing about Fred and Ben was their size: both were very heavy, big dudes. Fred had to be pushing 350 pounds, where Ben was probably hovering in the high 200 range.

Fred and Ben were shuffling along, just like me.

"Good morning," I shouted as they approached.

Both smiled and as we passed each other. Fred called, "What are you training for?"

I turned and screamed, "A long triathlon! What about you?"

Fred craned his neck back toward me and hollered, "A marathon, with my boy, here! December!"

And just like that, we lumbered past each other, going on our own paths. I found myself back in sissy land, crying and running. Two things about that little exchange brought me to welled-up scrunchy cry face.

First, Fred and Ben were two large people and I am no stranger to big people. They were out there *together*, making it happen, hobbling along, just as I was doing. My tears flowed from being an eyewitness to their mission and ultimate goal. To see and hear people vocalizing their crazy dreams is wonderful and affirming. People who are big, move slowly, and dream even bigger make me so happy!

The second remarkable thing was the moment when I shouted that I was training for my triathlon. I had said it few times out loud to anyone who cared to listen. But to literally scream it across a trail to complete strangers felt amazing.

I was crying for those reasons. I was crying because I was still "fat" according to all standards in this country. I was crying because on that day, I may have been any name someone called me—but I was mostly a girl who continued going and finished the morning with 11 miles in her shoes.

WORKING THROUGH INJURY

I am a massive klutz. I often fall off my bike and crush my hands and knees. I have scraped up my calves with chain bites. I do other things like wedging a sliver of laminate flooring under my thumbnail while cleaning up after the kids. I can get hurt anywhere: triathlon, cleaning or work, walking to the bathroom, tripping over a chicken wing, slipping in a puddle of someone else's sweat, doing the laundry, and there was that toenail incident in yoga class (all true).

Eight weeks before my second IRONMAN 70.3, I encountered either my own two feet (entirely possible) or roly pinecone.

Only the day before, the Expert and I had put down a sizeable bike ride, then a little 4-mile run. A bloody glorious brick where the sun was shining and I felt like a semireal triathlete. But Monday morning rolled in with a bang, and I ran out of the house a little too quickly toward the car.

I hit the ground, heard a snap, and glanced up to see the neighbor across the street staring at me. My work bag, my purse, and my keys were splayed across the yard. I was so stinking humiliated that I popped up like a gimpy jack-in-the-box and limped to the house. *Bollocks! My house key is in the yard!*

Immediately, my foot was throbbing. I rang the doorbell sixteen times before the Expert open the door and screamed, "*What* do you want? Good grief, Mere!"

"Let me in," I wailed, "I fell!" I was sobbing. "New Orleans!"

The Expert stared at me. The kids stared at me. I had fallen, then I had hobbled into the house, crying like a maniac. And the only significant thing I had to say was, "New Orleans." Crying about my upcoming 70.3 race.

Later that day, I learned that I broke the fifth metatarsal bone in my right foot. Oh, I broke it good, too. In two places. The man carrying the snazzy gray boot said something like, "Say hello to your little friend." I thought, *Say hello to my middle finger.* But I said nothing, I behaved, and I wore the boot outside the office, brandishing my crutches like a true champ. I was upset, but I was dealing. I called Gerry, who proceeded to talk in a string of appropriately timed expletives.

The eight-week countdown to my second IRONMAN 70.3 had *just* begun, and *I fell in my flipping yard. My yard!* And no training? I knew I would be seeing some depression and dark days.

Fast-forward eight weeks. I was up 15 (!) pounds and had lost every ounce of my endurance. At least, that was how I felt. I felt terrible. My food choices had been poor during the recovery period and the return to the gym and pool was less than pretty. I experienced four stages to my triathlon injury.

Over the ensuing years, I hurt my shoulder, fractured my tibia, and knotted up a zillion tendons, muscles, and more. Injury is part of sport. And when you get an injury, sometimes you have to go through the process of these four stages: grief, madness, coping, and retrieval.

Grief

Much as for a death, I mourned the demise of my second IRONMAN 70.3 dream. I sobbed at the thought of my running legs' melting down to squishy stumpy things, much like they had been two years earlier. I was forced to look at my rear end and invite more of its fat cell friends to leap upon it. I had ingrained my upcoming race in my skin and now that life was gone. Of course, that life was not gone. It was only temporarily unavailable. But loss, no matter how small, is still loss. I had to look my loss in the face, cry, and grieve it.

The more we practice the grief of the injury muscle, the more we can rebound from it. Injury—I'll repeat—is part of sport.

Madness

After I cried for three straight days, I went mad. I entered crazy land. All I heard were crazy voices: *How are you ever going to run again? You are going to become mentally unstable! What about your bicycle? Won't your bicycle be lonely? Will the gels in the cabinet actually go bad?*

I began to dream of nothing but running. I would run in my sleep and wake up whimpering from the pain. I would think about running at work. I would pack my cycling shoes for work, forgetting that Spin class was not on the list of acceptable behaviors for a newly broken metatarsal. The pure madness (insanity) then quickly turned to real madness (anger). I was mad, mad, and more mad.

Coping

After the grief and the madness, I began to cope. Notice I did not say that I began to "thrive." This stage was less insane, but it was merely manageable. I spent time coping with the fact that I could not run. I was dealing with my sadness for missing race day(s). I whined about missing my favorite cycling class. I learned new ways to get in some swimming (take off boot, limp to pool, get in carefully, and hope no one kicks me and breaks my foot in a third place).

Retrieval

The last stage of a triathlon injury is retrieval. Retrieval? What? Yes. Trying to *retrieve* muscle memory and retrieve the drive to get moving again. This is a big mental stage. Putting weight on the foot and trying to move normally was strange, so my retrieval stage consisted of trying to get things back to normal.

Retrieval was harder than the actual injury phase, because I had to stop comparing myself to . . . myself. I could not dwell on how much further along I was last year. I had to move on. Retrieve what I could, and get *back* to moving *forward*.

The biggest thing to remember about any injury is to follow your coach's, doctor's, and therapist's orders. Whatever you do, do *not* read online about your prognosis. Create your own prognosis (within reason) and allow your mind to heal your body. Continue to stay mentally positive and it will serve you well in the dark times. Time really does pass quickly, and you'll be back in the game before you realize it.

Looking back on the broken foot injury, however, so many years later, I can report that "this, too, passed" and I was fine. Sure, I experienced other injuries, and those, too, passed. One of the best things to do is keep perspective that time will heal the injury (most likely) and to not believe that it is the end of everything. Perspective becomes our friend—even when we don't want to hear it. We can figure out ways around the injury—even if we don't have a full recovery. Unless we are professional triathletes, it's really okay. Truly.

WORKING THROUGH BURNOUT

We often start the sport of triathlon like a love story—hot and heavy and nothing can be wrong with it. But like any relationship, having a healthy one with triathlon is important. Even the best relationships? Well, it's easy to get tired of the other person.

In other words, it *is* possible to tire of this amazing sport, the people in it, your swimsuit, bike, and shoes. The list is endless on the possibilities of joy—*and* burnout.

One of the things you can do to overcome burnout is to recognize that it exists. Many triathletes are floating down denial on this face. But burnout is real and it *will* impact you at some point in your triathlon journey.

Usually a nice step back—for a short time, a season or even a few years—is all you need to get back in the game. Also, it's possible to just move on after a season or two. Many of us get "the goody" out of the sport (e.g., we learn to workout, take care of ourselves, and achieve big goals), and we don't have a desire to continue doing triathlon. Guess what? That is okay, too!

You didn't sign a pact with the triathlon devil. And if you feel that way? Well, that's a sure sign that you need a break. Take one, do something else, and reassess. Remember: triathlon should *add* to your life—not take away from it.

DNS OR DNF: DID NOT START OR FINISH

The dreaded DNS and DNF—did not *start* and did not *finish* a race—well, both are likely to happen to you if you spend any time in this journey.

The DNS

With regard to *not starting* a race, I contend that this can be a great decision under certain circumstances. But how do we know that showing up and racing is the "right" call? In circumstances like this, I like to ask myself three questions:

How undertrained am I?

Notice this is not "Did I train enough?" (I mean, do we *ever* train perfectly?) By asking how much I am undertrained, I am considering whether I am rested from recovering from workouts, or rested from sheer missing of workouts. I am considering my base fitness. If you are slightly undertrained, that's okay. If you didn't bother to show up to the vast majority of your workouts, then that's a factor to consider.

Is my heart on fire for this race?

Undertraining might be (ever so slightly) overcome by the desire to do the race, and the mental fortitude and burning fire in the soul to finish. So, if you had a tough run of it, but your heart is on fire and you are determined to make it happen, this is a pretty big plus. However, if the circumstances leading up to the race have taken the air out of your balloon, then maybe it's not the right time.

What is the worst-case scenario?

With this question, I try to keep out the "really bad" worst case. I think more along the lines of surface-level worst case: *I will need to quit at the next aid station. I will have to do some walking on the run.* If the damage or potential worst case is relatively minor, then it might be something to overcome. However, being injured and risking further injury, missing out on a big family life-event, being undertrained and having *no* business tackling a race of that distance . . . those are all valid reasons for considering a DNS.

Will this race make me better, in some way, shape, or form?

Will racing improve your fitness, emotional state, heart, or soul? If the answer is no to any of the foregoing, then it's likely a prime candidate for a DNS. After all, we do this sport for the love, the benefits, and the memories. If none of those is good, then what's the point in showing up? Save the money and sleep in (this time).

The DNF

DNF ("did not finish") is perhaps the ickiest phrase in triathlon. The DNF is the dreaded result where something goes wrong and you're forced to drop out, whether you wanted to (think: uncooperative stomach, injury) or not (missed a time cutoff).

I have not DNFed a race (yet), but I have been *very close* in two of the biggest races of my life. I had a bad experience in one of them, where I wasn't sure whether I would make it, and my Garmin was dead, so I had no idea where I was, timing-wise. As a triathlon coach, I have had a few athletes DNF, and I know the heartbreak and devastation associated with it. First of all, it just sucks, and it's okay to be sad about it. But after wallowing for a day or two, realize that a DNF is simply a gift in disguise—a chance to improve your physical and mental game. Here's how to turn the crusty nugget of a DNF into gold.

Step 1: Realize you should be proud for starting.

You showed up to the race—that alone is a huge accomplishment. Think of all the training and dedication and hours that you put into getting there and putting yourself in the game on race day healthy and injury-free (or mostly injury-free). That's a victory in itself.

Step 2: Distinguish between what you could control on race day, and what you could not.

In my first IRONMAN, I had an acquaintance who was a fast racer, and he finished in fourteen hours and some change. (Of course, to me that *is* superfast, but he was more like an 11- or 12-hour guy.) What happened? He had not one, not two, but *four* flat tires on the course, which cost him more than two hours. He had to wait for assistance for the fourth, which took a massive chunk of time. You get my drift—if you showed up on race day as the best version of yourself and were ready to race, and then you had a mechanical, or a crash, or the weather was out of control and unforeseeably crazy, or something worse—you can't beat yourself up over that. Focus on what you could control on race day. If an unexpected event knocked you out, then breathe. What could you have done about that? Nothing.

Step 3: Grieve your loss.

I believe wholeheartedly in taking time to go through the emotions of what just happened. Give yourself time to be mad, cry, throw things, toss your bike down a mountain—a DNF is a complete *loss*. Acknowledge it as one. Missing out on hearing the words "You are an IRONMAN" or receiving your finisher's medal at your first race, while your whole family was there to support you—that is a *loss*, and you have the right to be sad and mourn it. Give yourself some time to do that. I hate when I am in the middle of a personal or triathlon crisis hearing the phrase "It could be worse." Of course it can *always* be worse! That doesn't mean that you aren't in the middle of pain. Right now, the truth and reality after a DNF *hurts* and stings. Grieve. Have your time of madness, and after you have sufficiently done these things, only then can you figure out how to move on.

Step 4: Evaluate what actually happened on race day.

What story is *your* story of the DNF? What are the lessons to be learned? What do you want next, if anything?

I encourage my athletes to write a race report, even if just for themselves. The emotions, the facts, and everything in between should be included so that they can really analyze what went wrong and what went right—where they could change things if they had a redo. Race day may have included curve balls that caused or contributed to your DNF. Race day may have presented challenges that you weren't prepared to handle—physically or emotionally or gear-wise. It could be that you just weren't prepared for that particular type or distance race on that day, in that particular time in your life. (Note: It doesn't mean that you won't ever be.) Accept the truth of the race—whatever that may be—and then forgive whatever may have happened (the weather, your bicycle, yourself) and prepare to, in the words of *Frozen*, let it go. Be kind to yourself. It won't be instant. But it's part of the process.

TRIATHLON AS HEALING

I urge you to remember this phrase:

> "The bad things will not define me.
> The bad people will not discourage me."

Sometimes I use triathlon as a demon exorciser, a healthy power. Sometimes I run so far and swim so many laps, I forget how to even count.

One particular swim comes to mind. After a hideous day, I started off the swim *mad as all hell* from work. I was absolutely fuming as I took off for the first 300-meter warm-up. I swam and swam and swam. I got madder, then I got faster. Then, I started to smolder instead of just fume. I swam more: 200s. 300s. 50s. 100s. 400s. I prayed. I cried a little, inside my goggles.

I swam for almost two straight hours. I swam until my shoulders and back ached more than my brain. I swam until my anger was washed away with the chlorine and nothing but a dull, throbbing memory of the day remained. I wandered to the shower exhausted, and as I rinsed off my suit and the chlorine, I began crying again. And I thanked God for triathlon.

That night, I walked in the door with wet hair. I hugged the Expert. I cuddled my kids. I ate a giant bowl of spaghetti and two Reese's cups. I did not feel guilty. I felt healed. I knew that another day of worries would come (in approximately 12 hours).

Triathlon has changed me.

During that one swim workout, I was able to remember to say: *The bad things will not define me. The bad people will not discourage me.* I can honestly say that I was shown the grace of God through a simple, yet very long, swim.

Over the years, I have found long bike rides to do the same. I have found runs to bring on tears and healing. I have also learned that triathlon is not the center of the universe for me. I have learned that it became the impetus for me to *find* myself.

I wish the same for you.

Find the run. Find the swim. Find your quiet place. Hold onto those precious, quiet, and difficult training moments. You will find that sometimes the most painful workouts, and the most hideous race photos, are often the most healing.

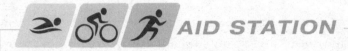

AID STATION

THE GREATEST RIDE I NEVER HAD

I was about three years into triathlon training and I was obsessed with everything swim, bike, and run. I loved all the things about the sport and I was growing and learning more every single day. I stuck to my training plan with a crazy rigidity that I didn't know I had inside me. All good things.

At the same time, my personal life, marriage, and job were suffering. My relationship with my young children was difficult—in the sense that I wasn't doing the best job of being present for them. I would go out and run or ride long, and I would be present in body when I returned—but I could barely keep my eyes open. I still contend that I am a better mother, wife, and employee when I am training, but sometimes that long-distance training takes a toll unlike any other.

That is part of the triathlon training, I am convinced—that we learn to manage our lives in new ways. I have noticed those who have longevity in this sport as age-groupers identify and live in that special world that encompasses family, life, fun, and triathlon. Those I have seen who fizzle out? Well, the fizzle often comes when triathlon becomes life, and then life starts to implode.

So, I was training for my first IRONMAN in 2013 and I had a 100-mile ride on the books for the day. I was scheduled for what I remember to be four of five 100-milers before the race, so this was one of those critical rides. I was woken up by my almost-four-year-old around 4:30 a.m., about 30 minutes before I was supposed to wake up (the worst). She crawled into bed with me, grabbed her blankie, and started sucking her thumb. For a moment, I was so aggravated—only thirty minutes left to

continues

continued

sleep and she gets me up!—but then I closed my eyes and felt a deep sense of sadness for my thought: *What is wrong with me?* Then, I fell into the rhythm of her thumb-sucking, her little breaths, her sweet still-a-baby-but-not-a-baby smell. I reached over, clicked off my alarm, and went back to sleep.

A couple of hours later, I woke up with her. My husband made breakfast. We drank coffee. I brushed my teeth, but that was all. I watched movies all day in bed in my pj's with the kids. I read an entire book before the sun went down. I didn't ride—at all—not even the trainer. We had a full-family lazy day.

Five years and four IRONMAN races later, of all the amazing memories from triathlon and racing, I must admit that I cherish that day with my family more than any other day of racing. That's not to say that training is always worth skipping—I am not saying to be a slacker. But sometimes those "big workout days" are better spent in another arena of our lives. As long as we are alive, there will always be another workout, another race—even if we are injured, old, slow, or sick. However, life and precious time with those people we love? There are no guarantees we will have that forever—not in those exact moments. When those moments present themselves, let the rest go—be present, be brave, and be thankful. You won't regret it.

14 LOST IN TRANSITION

Time to "transition" back to triathlon and racing. And up next is the topic of transition.

Transition was a confusing topic for me when I started thinking about triathlon. Everyone was talking about "T1" and "T2" and I had no earthly idea what those meant. *Were they something to do with a toilet? I need to do a T1?* Sometimes. But really, *transition* means two things.

First, *transition* as a *noun*: the place where you store your bike (and other stuff) during a race. This location is usually a large, open area with metal racks for the bikes. You will likely have an assigned space on the rack for your bike, and a space under your bike to place your triathlon "things."

Second, *transition* as a *verb*: the action of moving between the sports of swim to bike, and then bike to run. You transition from the swim to the bike. Then, you transition from the bike to the run.

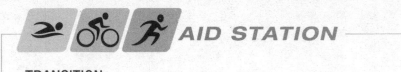

TRANSITION

In summary, all you need to remember is to ask yourself: am I wearing what I should be wearing for the sport I am about to do?

Goggles go with swim. Helmet goes with bike. Really, transition is like a preschool game of *Memory*. But the problem in the middle of a race is, you are actually thinking like a cranky preschooler—so remembering to wear the proper gear is more challenging than you might imagine.

The best advice I have about transition in your first few races is: *take your time*. I know it is counterintuitive to "take your time" in a *race*. But making a strong exit from transition is more beneficial than making a fast (and potentially clumsy) exit—wearing your helmet on the run.

In a later section in this book covering race day, I will go into detail about the things you need for your race and how to set up your transition area—but for now, here's a quick overview of transition—the noun *and* the verb.

T1

T1 is the transition from the end of the swim to the bike.

When you are finishing up your swim, that is the time you begin to think of your transition to the bike: *Where is my bike? Repeat the order of your transition in your head: helmet, glasses, shoes, race number belt with number turned to the back* (or whatever order you choose). This will make a smooth transition onto the bike.

Again, as a beginner, take your time in both transitions, especially in your first race. Yes, this whole thing is about *racing*. But you don't want to come barreling out of transition without your helmet and get disqualified. Take a moment to gather your composure, and ensure that you have all your gear (and wits) about you. Sometimes it helps to catch your breath.

As I am coming out of the water, I usually take off my goggles and swim cap. If you are wearing a wetsuit, you can pull the wetsuit down to your waist as you are coming out of the water. Races will have "strippers" (woo-hoo! Triathlon is *awesome*! Okay, not *those* kind of strippers . . .)—volunteers who help *strip* off your wetsuit near the swim exit. You sit on your bum, lean back, and they *riiiiiip* your wetsuit from your body. Fun times! Let them help you; it's much easier that way!

Once you are in your transition area, it might help to have an extra bottle of water to spray off your feet and eyes (especially after a saltwater swim). Usually you will have mud, sand, or grass on your feet from the run *into* T1 after the swim—hence the handiness of the water bottle. Sometimes the race director will have a baby pool to step into to clean your feet, but sometimes you may overlook the pool or it may be crowded (or dirtier than your feet!). I have found this water bottle tip to be great advice! I love to rinse and quickly wipe my feet before putting on my bike shoes.

In shorter races, I do not wear socks on the bike because my feet are wet and wet socks are frustrating. By the time I run, I am usually dry enough to put on socks. Or I will wear socks on the bike and then put on fresh socks before the run. However, this is a matter of personal preference—do what works for you! Once you are helmeted, race number clipped on (use a race number belt, described later) and ready, you can head out to bike. (And no, you do not use a towel to *dry off* your body before getting on the bike. Crazy, I know. Get on that bike sopping wet—you'll survive, I promise!)

You must roll (not ride) your bike out of the transition area. There will usually be a banner or a sign: BIKE EXIT. Head that way, walking alongside your bike, but do not get *on* your bike until after the mount line.

Mount line? What?

Before the race, make note of where the "Bike Mount" line is. Most races have an actual line of tape or paint placed on the ground right outside of the transition bike exit. Sometimes they designate it with construction cones or a sign: MOUNT HERE. Regardless of what the line is—it is only *after* this line or designated area that you are allowed to get on your bike and ride. Do *not* mount your bike before this line or you can get disqualified. Usually the volunteers are very good about letting you know (screaming, if necessary) where to be and when to get on your bike.

The best practice is to roll your bike past this line and over to the right side (to make room for those who are flying out of transition). Clip safely into your pedals if you have clipless ones and pedal off for the bike leg.

As a beginner, the race will be confusing enough. If you get nervous or confused, just move to the right side of the course (out of everyone's way) and gain your composure before moving again. But always get yourself to the right—don't just stop in the middle of *anywhere* in a race.

T2

T2 is the second transition when you finish the bike and begin your run.

Much like the way *out* of transition—you do not ride *into* transition, either. You must walk and roll your bike back to your spot. As you are riding your bike toward T2, you will see a "Bike Dismount" or "Dismount Here" line. You must dismount your bike *before* this line. Sometimes the dismount line is the same as the mount line; sometimes they are in two different places—just check before you begin the race.

If you are shaky on the dismount, slow down well in advance of transition and pull to the right and take your time dismounting. Once you are off your bike, roll your bike to your transition spot and rack your bike.

At this point, you are ready to take off your helmet and bike shoes and get ready to run. Turn your race number to the front, find your hat or visor, slip on those running shoes (and socks if you are like me and bike without), and get moving!

As the Expert says when he is spectating my races: "Run and done!" That is my favorite mantra after the bike. I repeat it often: *Run and done and run and done and run and done and run . . .*

T3

Fooled you. No such thing as T3.

Well, actually there is. T3 is the time after the race where you wander around aimlessly looking for snacks and your people.

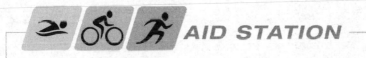

AID STATION

Practice your transitions before race day. You will look funny in your driveway, but who cares? Better for your neighbors to think you are nuts than your fellow triathletes.

15 RACE PREPARATION AND RACE DAY

I CAN PROMISE YOU: YOU *WILL*, AT SOME POINT, ENCOUNTER SOME crazy triathlon things on race day (almost every triathlete, new or seasoned, has). However, proper preparation for your race can certainly help alleviate some of the nuttiness that can come your way.

THE TAPER

One to two weeks before any longer distance race (Olympic and longer) comes the taper.

The idea behind the taper is that you have put in the miles and you are ready, but you must give the body time to recover and rest prior to the big day. The purpose of the taper is to allow your body to recover from the pounding and to restore the glycogen levels in your bloodstream and liver. A very common mistake is to show up for races tired. The point of the taper is to put *pop* back into your legs and your mind.

Shorter distance races (sprint distance) don't necessarily require a "real" taper. But you do need rest, regardless. You can reduce the quantity of your workouts the week before and just stretch, swim and stay loosey-goosey. Practice your mental feats of strength during this time!

THE WEEK BEFORE: PRE-RACE!
Pre-race Rest

The amount of pre-race rest you require depends also on distance of race. Of course, you need a good night's sleep, but I'm talking about training *rest*. Take the time to reduce your training a little and rest at night and during the day.

Pre-race Nutrition

In the days leading up to race day, you may want to up your carbohydrates a *little*. Gone are the days of super carb loading from a nutritional stand-point. Even still, this advice is really only important for longer-distance races. Do not load up on pasta before your two-hour race (or perhaps any time). You don't need it, and it will just make you feel icky.

Pre-race Hydration

Hydration is extremely important during training and leading up to race day. You must, however, be careful that you are taking in the right amount of water, sodium, and potassium. Drinking so much water that it dilutes the sodium in your blood can, in extreme cases, be fatal. Keeping the right electrolyte balance is important, but again, it is more important in the longer distance races. See Chapter 11 for more.

All the Things

I highly recommend making a list of the things you need for the race and checking it twice, Santa-like. You need things before the race, during, and after. Practice your transitions and take note of your list! For your first race, pack your bag several days before. Unpack it and practice your transitions, then repack it. This will ensure that you have everything you need and get you some extra transition practice.

The following is a great starting point for your first or next triathlon checklist.

Pre-race

Tri kit/tri suit

Race bag/gym bag

Pre-race snack

Helmet and bike numbers (affixed to helmet and bike)

Sunscreen (only after you have been marked with race number)

Swim

Goggles and swim cap

Extra pair of goggles

Wetsuit (if needed)

Lubricant (for under your arms or to prevent wetsuit chafing)

T1/Bike

Bike!

Helmet

Cycling shoes

Towel or transition mat

Water bottle (to rinse feet after swim)

Small towel (to wipe feet before putting on your shoes)

Water bottles for bike

Socks

Sunglasses

Nutrition to consume on the bike

Heart rate monitor/GPS watch

Bike tools (tube, CO_2, tire levers)

T2/Run

Running shoes

Race number belt with race number attached

Large resealable plastic bag (in case it rains, you can put your running shoes in here to keep them semidry at least for the start)

Hat/visor

Socks

Hydration belt (optional; usually for longer distances)

Nutrition

Post-race

Change of clothes and shoes

A smile

A GPS to find the post-race snacks

Mental Preparation

Like everything else in triathlon, race day preparation is very much part of the mental game. Gerry told me, "I will go through the whole race in my mind in race week and through my training. I don't visualize the *perfect* race. Instead, I visualize things that could go wrong and I picture myself dealing with these issues calmly and confidently. I remind myself of the work I have done. I go back through my logs and think about the 'deposits' I have made. I bring my checkbook on race day, and I write the check."

[I laughed at him here.]

Mike Reilly, the announcer and "Voice of Ironman," on race morning says: "There is only one thing you can control today—and that is your attitude."[1]

Take each leg of the race as it comes—one bite of the elephant at a time. (I don't know why anyone is eating elephants, but that's what triathlon essentially is.) When you are thinking about swimming, you should be swimming. When you are thinking about riding, you should be on your bike. Don't worry about the run until and unless you are running—even then, don't worry. Just run or walk—keep moving forward.

Be present in the moment with what you are doing, and don't worry about what is in the past—or what is next.

Truly having a good attitude and celebrating what your amazing body *can do*, will carry you from the start to finish with a smile on your face—no matter how hard it gets on the course.

Race Day Clothing

Listen up, ladies. I talked about this earlier and I'm going to talk about it again. You want to get a triathlon suit or "kit" for your race. End of story.

You have the option to go with a triathlon-like alternative, but you may *not* deviate far. This is Newbie Rule 101. Trust me on this. And don't e-mail me asking whether you can change clothes in transition—I will not write you back because this has been explained. Do. Not. Show. Your. Goodies. In. Transition. Ever.

THE DAY BEFORE THE RACE
Packet Pickup

Not all races will have athlete check-in or bike check the day prior to the race. However, many of the big races *do*. Read your registration and rules and know the schedule.

When you pick up your race packet, ensure that you have everything you need *in* the packet. Most races include a swim cap, race number, helmet and bike sticker, and timing chip with a strap for your ankle. Do not leave the race venue until you have all the parts to your packet. I learned this lesson the way I learn most of my lessons (a.k.a. the hard way). I drove an hour to the race venue (with kids!) only to get home and realize that I had forgotten my timing chip. Back to the race venue (with kids!) I went.

Some packets will include number "tattoos" for you to apply to your arms and legs. Do not apply these until race morning—or you can put them on right before bed. They usually do survive a night's sleep. Read the instructions to the race tattoos carefully and do not apply your lotion or sunscreen until *after* you have affixed the numbers.

Bike Check-in

Confirm that your bike and components (spare tire tube, bike bag, lubed bike, pumped tires) are all in order *before* bike check-in. Do not place your water bottles or your bike "accessories" (helmet, shoes) in transition if you check your bike the day before the race. You want to wait until the morning of the race to *bring* all these items.

The race officials will let you into transition on the morning of the race, so you will be able to reevaluate your bike and tires, bring all your gear, and set up your transition area before the race start. You may be required to affix the bike number to your bike before checking it, but usually that's all that is required before checking the bike.

RACE BREAK

A FIRST OLYMPIC DISTANCE

St. Anthony's Triathlon, May 1, 2011
1.5K (0.9-mile) swim
40K (24.8-mile) bike
10K (6.2-mile) run

The Expert and I woke up at 4:15 a.m. I did not sleep well, but with the nerves, I had not really expected to. We arrived at the race venue and set up our transition area.

Swim

I was in the sixth wave start. My fellow green swim-capped Athenas and I were all together. It was a beach start, meaning we were all corralled in a place on the beach, and when the buzzer went off, we would run

continues

continued

toward the water and begin the swim. The Expert was on the beach, his wave leaving much later. He waved at me and I waved back. So many waves.

The buzzer went off, and the other ladies took off running at the speed of light. *Zoom!* into the water. I jogged a little slower and was one of the last ones in. The swim was fabulous. No panic, no freak-outs, and I was stoked.

I took my sweet time in T1. I went to the bathroom. I wandered around my bike a little. I was slow. I was okay with that.

Bike

I was most concerned with two things about the bike portion of the race: mount and dismount. A small miracle happened for me: both were nonissues.

The bike course was amazing—flat, fast, and humbling. I passed only twenty or so riders during the entire 24 miles. I was passed by hundreds and hundreds. I was riding at a good clip, but I might as well have been moving backward.

We all wore our age on our left calf, written with Sharpie. My bike buddy and I rode most of the race together, switching back and forth. Later, as we racked our bikes for the run, I found out that this amazing woman was eighty-year-old Sister Madonna Buder, a multiple finisher at the world's biggest race, the IRONMAN World Championship in Kona. She had a finish time of 3:20:50 at St. Anthony's, beating me by a solid three minutes.

Run

T2 was a little faster than T1. I dashed out of the transition area with fury (without my helmet, I'm proud to add). Okay, so that statement is not accurate. I trotted out slowly and carefully, knowing full well that 6.2 miles is no joke, especially after a swim and a bike. I didn't want to lose any of my precious steam.

The run course was an "out and back" format. The Expert had started his race about forty-five minutes after me, so I knew I would see him at

continues

continued

some point on the course. As I had 1.2 miles left on the run, the Expert and I passed each other. I was so happy to see him, and I would later learn that seeing a friend on the course always makes the pain stop, even if only for a few seconds.

I was incredibly slow. My right calf was still a mess from my low-speed tip-over on the bike that I had experienced at a stoplight the day before. Most people must have thought I had fallen on the course, because I received many, many "Way to go" comments and "Just keep going" shouts. I may have been moving ridiculously slow, but really, I had never felt so good in a run—well, until I reached Mile 5.5. My calves started cramping, the sun was beating down, and I was praying for the end of the race. I could hear drums in the distance. *The finish line!* I brought the run home in 1:18:59 (12:44 pace), and as I turned into the final stretch, the street was lined with cheering people, happy faces, and I felt blessed to the point of tears.

The goal was accomplished . . . and felt amazing! But as I crossed the finish, I gained much more than just a personal pat on the back. I gained a true sense of thankfulness and humility, and I stand in absolute awe of all the amazing athletes who compete in this sport.

Never once during the race did I have a single negative thought, like *I can't* or *This is impossible*. Not once. That in itself is a miracle.

Every time I began to hurt or feel some negative clouds rolling in, I closed my eyes and remembered to be thankful, to consider the able body I had. My official race time was 3:22:34, with the longest T1 time in the history of man.

RACE DAY

The Morning of Your Race

Practice your positive race visualizations as you get ready for the race. Make sure you get your first poop in, er, out—ideally before you leave the hotel or house. Coffee is good for this. You'll be glad you did. Trying to poop in a Porta-Potty with twenty people in line behind you is less than ideal.

Eat well in advance of the race (2 to 3 hours). Do not fret too much about your nutrition on a sprint distance race. Eat something reasonably substantial for breakfast, but low in grease and fiber. Think: bagel with peanut butter, oatmeal with nuts. Remember the rule: do not try anything new. This includes food. I would suggest eating what you did on days before you went on your longer bike rides. You know that agrees with you. Plus, your stomach may be nervous.

If you anticipate being on the race course for more than two hours, then consider packing a gel or a snack to eat on the bicycle leg. Typically, you will not need nutrition on a short race. However, if you are a big girl and are moving slower than others, pack some nutrition. Trust me. I eat *something* on *all* distance races. I may have a gel on the bike and another one at the start of the run. Triathlon is tough enough without the dreaded bonk. This is your race, so do what is best for *you*.

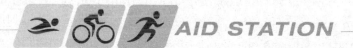 **AID STATION**

"THE BONK"

A bonk is also known as "hitting the wall" and pretty much feels like absolute crap murder poop face pain. When your body uses its glycogen stores, you will "bonk"—you will know the bonk when it happens, but you really don't ever want it to happen. In other words, you will want to make sure that you eat/nutritionize yourself for anything over an hour to an hour and a half of exercise or racing. Your body, for the most part, can store up to this much glycogen for use without supplementation. Of course, there are exceptions to every rule, and fat-adapted athletes or those in ketosis are exceptions (curious? Ask Google). Generally speaking, though, you can avoid the bonk by eating and ingesting calories at the right times.

Something about a true "bonk" will rip a person apart. The triathlon bonk is caused by a depletion of glycogen storage in the body. Usually, you bonk because you are under-fueled and have depleted your sugar/carb stores.

Setting Up Your Transition Area

Once you have your race packet, numbers, bike, and timing chip, you are ready to head into transition to set up.

Timing Chip

Your timing chip will most likely be on an ankle strap. The timing chip registers your placement on the course (depending on the race), or at a minimum, when you cross the finish line. You wear it for the entire race.

You can put this on immediately or wait until after you put on your wetsuit (if needed). I recommend putting it on as soon as possible, so it is not lost in the transition setup. You can always remove it to pull on your wetsuit.

Find Your Spot

You will likely have either an assigned spot in transition or an assigned area based on your race number. Some races are just a first-come, first-serve transition, so you can place your bike anywhere you would like. You will "rack" your bike, usually by lifting the rear of your bike and hooking the front of your saddle on the rack. If this is confusing now, it won't be on race morning. Just look around you and you will see how the bikes are resting by their saddles.

Of course, it varies by race, but usually there will be rows and rows of metal racks in transition. Depending on the size of the rack in each row, you may have fifteen to one hundred bikes on "your" row. As you rack your bike, remember to stagger it with your neighbor's bike. For example, if your transition neighbor's front wheel is facing one way, you should rack your bike the *opposite* way—with your *rear* wheel next to her *front* wheel. This prevents handlebars from getting tangled up when removing the bikes from the rack in T1, and also when you are re-racking your bike in T2.

Set Up Your Area

Remember to be courteous with your transition area. Gerry says, "It is important to be respectful. Your transition area should be no larger than a small towel—*not* a small town. The key to transition—both setting up the area and executing T1 and T2—is practicing the ritual and finding a sequence. Once you find this sequence, then you should do it the same way every time. To have the consistency, you must practice so it's second nature."

There are a zillion options about where to place your transition area *stuff*. But the space to the left of the front wheel makes the most practical sense, after all. In T1, you will stand at your bike, put on your shoes, helmet, and so on, and then unhook your bike and roll it toward the BIKE OUT banner. If your stuff is at your *rear* wheel—theoretically, you'd have to either squeeze your bike *under* the rack (which is impossible if you are tall and have a large bike), or walk around the transition rack to the other side.

So, go with the left of your front wheel.

- No matter the location of your transition area, keep it in line with your neighbors' setup. Roll with the punches. If you are the first one there setting up, go with the left of your front wheel, because that makes the most sense, and that's how it's done in the big races.
- Keep your transition area small. Be courteous of others! A bath towel (folded in half!) or mat sold specifically for transitions is a perfect size for your area. Stay on your towel area, and your neighbors will be grateful.
- If you have a backpack in transition with you, find a friend or family member (who is not racing) to hold it during the race. If you are racing alone, squeeze your bag under your bike or against the transition area fence (if allowed—some races do not, and it's often against USAT rules).
- Don't be nosy. Mind your own business and don't tell others what to do or what *not* to do in transition. Unless they're infringing on your transition area real estate, fumbling with your stuff or your bike, just take a deep breath and let it go.

When you arrive at the race on race morning, you will have a certain period of time before transition closes. During this time, you should set up your area. First, lay your transition mat or folded towel on the ground.

Then, place the items you need for the bike and the run on the towel *in the same manner that you practiced beforehand* during your training. Remember: you should not try anything new on race day and this includes your transition area setup.

I like to place my cycling shoes on the front left of the mat or towel. Next to the shoes, I have my water bottle (to spray my feet), a small washcloth or towel, and my helmet, which is upside down and precisely turned around so I can put it directly on my head. Inside my helmet, I have my sunglasses and race number belt. Some people like to put their helmet on the handlebars of their bike—this is a good reminder to put your helmet on—because you can't roll your bike without touching the helmet. My order for T1 is: sunglasses, helmet, race number belt (number to the rear), spray feet, wipe feet, shoes, and go. It does not matter what order you choose; just find your order and keep it consistent.

If you wear a wetsuit in the swim, you will want to roll it up or fold it as you run into T1 and place it neatly under your bike, or behind your towel.

To the rear of my cycling gear on the mat, I have my T2 gear: my running shoes on the rear left of the mat, with one sock inside of each shoe. To the right, I have my visor and my handheld water bottle or Fuel Belt.

As I come into T2, I rack my bike, unstrap my helmet, and put my helmet on the seat of my bike. Then, I slip off my cycling shoes and place them on the front of the mat. I slip *on* my socks, my running shoes, and my visor, and a Fuel Belt or handheld bottle, and I run out.

Have Your Bike in Gear

Your bike should be in the gear easiest for you to mount when coming out of transition. Don't forget to check this on race morning—trying to pedal when you're in the hardest gear is not only tough, but you might topple over.

Additionally, ensure that you have bar caps on the ends of your handlebars on a road bike before you check your bike into transition. Sometimes these plugs may fall out—and if you don't have your handlebar ends plugged, you can't race. After all, you don't want to fall during a race and gore your cycling neighbor.

Wetsuit

Only after your transition area is set up, need you worry about your wetsuit. If you are wearing a wetsuit for the swim portion, do *not* put the suit on an *hour* beforehand. I recommend putting it on, only waist high, twenty minutes before the race starts and pulling it up over your arms and zipping up only five to ten minutes before your wave takes off. (Otherwise, you can run the risk of overheating. Of course, if it's freezing outside, ignore everything I just wrote and do whatever you need to do to stay warm.) Do not forget your timing chip! You will need to take it off or wait to put on the timing chip until after you are wearing the suit.

THE HOUR BEFORE

Transition will close about an hour before your race start, leaving you with an hour to panic and wander around aimlessly, muttering things like *Why did I sign up for this?*

DON'T FORGET!

Make sure you have your swim cap and goggles when you leave transition. Once transition is "closed," it's really closed! I tuck my goggles and cap into my sports bra so I don't leave them behind, or put them down somewhere.

Depending on your personality, you should find the best way for *you* to cope with this extra time before the race. Whatever you do, do *not* look at the other athletes and start comparing yourself to them. There will be athletes like Frank McHotBod and Sally O'FastLegs. Ignore them and concentrate on the hard work that you have done to prepare.

The Expert likes to get in the water and warm up before a race. I like to find a place away from the crowd and separate myself from the hoopla. Depending on the race course setup (and outside temperatures), it may be a good idea to get in the water if you can. Personally, I get in the water to pee. I'm sorry, but that's what 99 percent of everyone is doing in the water during warm-up. Just embrace the pee water and you'll be okay.

THE FINAL FEW MINUTES

As you stand at the swim wave start with your new race swim cap on your head and your goggles pulled down over your eyes, take a look around you.

Then, take a deep breath.

Remember: while you are taking part in a competition, *competing* is not the main goal here. Remember that this race is the start of something wonderful in your life. Look at the others around you, but do *not* compare yourself to them. Look at your fellow racers with the realization that they, too, are nervous and anxious about *their race*. Remember that this is *your* race. Be thankful.

Take another deep breath.

Look to the sky. Say "thank you" to your God for letting you stand on that beach, dock, boat, deck, or grass. Embrace a feeling of gratitude and thankfulness as the national anthem is played (or if it's not your country's anthem, hum your own and be thankful anyway). Be humbled by your working body, your strong body that is going to get you across the finish line. Be thankful that you had the opportunity to train for the race. Realize that you have worked hard and you are ready for it. Thank your body for the hard work it is about to take on. Thank your mind for believing in *you*. Thank your soul for carrying the dream through.

Take another deep breath.

Carry the feeling of gratefulness during your entire race. Be strong between your ears, and that will keep your body strong. When you feel that you can't go on, then tell yourself, *Just keep moving forward* or use a mantra that you have used in training. Tell yourself, *I got this. I am ready.*

Take another deep breath. Because this is your day. You're here. Now, have fun!

16 TO LONG-DISTANCE TRIATHLON AND BEYOND

AFTER FINISHING ST. ANTHONY'S (AND NOT FINISHING LAST), I thought I would be feeling d-o-n-e and completely satisfied. Don't get me wrong, I was stoked to have finished that race.

I had not told anyone at this point, but two months *before* St. Anthony's, I had already registered for the next big thing. Two months before being certain that I could even *finish* an *Olympic* distance, I registered for a semicrazy goal race.

An IRONMAN 70.3 Miami would take place six months after St. Anthony's. The 70.3 is a race distance consisting of a 1.2-mile swim, 56-mile bike, and a half marathon. Pretty close to *double* the distance I had just completed. I was certain that Gerry would faint with exhaustion and shred his clothes in horror to train me to 70.3. (He didn't.)

Six months later, I finished my first IRONMAN 70.3. Less than two years after that, I finished my first IRONMAN—a race of a 2.4-mile swim, 112-mile bike, and 26.2-mile run. The official crazy had taken hold—as I went on to do three more, and who knows how many I'll actually finish before the End of Days.

Long-distance triathlon is way beyond the scope of this book, but I know that if you are like me—you have a sparkle in your eye and maybe a secret dream about finishing a 70.3 longer one or hearing those words "You are an IRONMAN." I get it, so I will talk about it (briefly).

SET THE DREAM INTO MOTION

If this is a thing you want, then go ahead and admit it. It's dumb to pretend you don't want something if you do. I am giving you a permission slip: YOU, *henceforth, have permission to want this crazy thing.*

Before You Register

We can all get mouse-happy with our little registration finger and register before it's really time to jump up in distances. Fear of missing out (FOMO) is a very real and dangerous thing in triathlon. Learn to realize that FOMO is okay. Have it sometimes.

Find a triathlon mentor—someone who will shoot you straight, encourage you where needed, but also level with you. If someone asks me for my honest opinion about his or her ability to move on a 70.3 or 140.6, I will give it. Otherwise, I will keep my mouth shut. But finding someone who will give you the truth—and not just feed the FOMO—is important.

Make sure that your family is on board. You will need its support. It's hard enough with undying support—without *any*? It truly is a disaster.

Ensure that you have adequate time to build the distance, the endurance base you *must* have for long-distance racing, and hire a coach if you can—at a minimum, get a solid training plan. For me, I think a coach is the best money spent for the first long-distance race. Just get a good coach—ask around, and don't be a lemming with your coach choice—find the person who fits *you*—not just the person who all your friends are flocking to.

Put in the Work

A 70.3 and beyond is a shitton of work. Let me repeat—if you are thrilled about registering and training with your friends, but you aren't into the work part . . . then, long-distance racing is not for you. It is hard work. It takes time. The time commitment for a 70.3 is conservatively twelve hours a week, not counting travel time and maintenance and the like. For an IRONMAN or 140.6? You can look at twenty-five hours easily and beyond—do you have time for another job? Because that's what it will take.

You need to have the fire burning in you that will fuel the work. Because the work becomes very real. Can you do it? Absolutely, but you must not only want to have the finish, you must also crave the work (and the boredom that goes along with it). Long-distance racing requires long-distance training—hours and hours of repetitive and boring work. If you can't stand to do the same thing for more than thirty minutes? It might make you insane.

None of this is to discourage you from long-distance. You can find a million people out there who will tell you, *"Do it!"* That's not hard to find—the triathlon FOMO instigators. What is hard is to find someone who will level with you, tell you the truth—and explain how much time, commitment, energy, and trauma it might be. That's me. That's a tri mentor. That's a coach.

Is it worth it? *That's up to you.*

Is the dream worth it? *Also up to you.*

If it is—go get it.

ON RACE DAY

There is one secret to long-distance racing, provided you have trained appropriately, are healthy, and have done all the things to put yourself in the best position possible.

The Secret: You must believe you will finish—no room for doubt whatsoever. Believe, and you are halfway there. This sense of belief must be automatic, unwavering, and, yes—like everything else in triathlon—requires training.

Next, like any other race—you must move forward all day long. Forward is a pace. Slow and steady doesn't win IRONMAN or 70.3, but it gets you to the finish—which is likely what you are after.

Sure, it might be a tooth-and-nail-fought almost-not-finish finish, sometimes within minutes of the end of the whole race. But you know what they call a C student who passes the bar exam by one point? A lawyer.

Same with an almost not-finisher-finisher—a finisher.

AFTER THE LETDOWN

After any big race—an IRONMAN or your first tri—there may be an emotional, spiritual, and physical letdown after it is complete. Let me rephrase—there *will* be a letdown.

There are many psychological and physiological reasons for this response, but I simply remind my athletes that it is coming. At some point, you will crash—and everyone handles it differently. I think that simply being prepared that the post-race blues is coming is the only thing we can do. To understand that your body, heart, and soul (and family) likely need a transition period of rest—and then to simply honor that need—will expedite the movement through the not-so-fun phase.

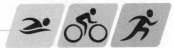

THE IRONMAN 70.3 MIAMI RACE REPORT

We arrived at the race venue about 5:15 a.m. The rain was pouring. Pouring. Pouring. We parked about 12,000 miles from transition.

Gerry called me. I knew who was calling without even looking at the phone. Only two crazy people could be calling me at that hour. And I had already talked to my dad for the early-morning pep talk. I answered.

continues

continued

Swim Start

I do not remember doing so, but I must have unpacked my stuff and set up my transition area. I remember the Expert pumped my tires. I was thankful for that. No way my hands could have worked. My transition area was ready, probably from no help of my own.

The Expert and I wandered to the swim start about 5:50 a.m. The rain continued to mercilessly come down, and we began to get cold. In Miami? Cold? Ridiculous. We found a place under a tree to sit, but the mean tree just poured fat, sloppy rain on us. Finally, I slapped on my swim cap just to keep my head warm. That worked a little.

"What have you gotten us into?" the Expert asked me.

"I don't want to talk about it," I said.

The sun appeared to come up, but only because the sky brightened. There was no actual sighting of said sun. About 7:30-ish, the first starting gun went off. The swim was set up like an evil triangle. A triangle that started with a jump off a dock, a swim out, and tread water until the gun started.

I was in Wave 9. The Expert was in Wave 15, I think. I kissed the Expert and waddled off in the rain to find my people. I did not go far, however, before I slipped one more time on the pavement. I did not fall, but as I was cursing, I had to dodge a falling age grouper as he hit the pavement.

This race is already sheer carnage, I thought.

I was pretty impressed with the wave organization. I followed a person waving a sign that said "Female 30–34" and had a silver swim cap attached to it. That was my wave! My wave! I looked around at my fellow silver caps. Unlike local races, there were no Average Janes. In local races, where I can race Athena, I felt a little more in place. Here? There were no Athenas in sight. In fact, there were no women who were within 15 pounds of Athena.

Where are the other little chubby girls? I thought. This was 2011 and triathlon was not nearly as diverse as it is now (even though it still needs work)—but I was seriously the only not-so-triathlete-looking woman on the course.

In that moment, I felt a little sick. *Had I had bitten off more than I could chew? Was I overconfident? Was I clinically insane?* The silver

continues

continued

caps inched our way down to the dock. I pulled my goggles down over my eyes.

Another starting gun and the wave ahead, the pink caps, took off. The silver caps all walked to the edge of the dock and we jumped in the water. I swam out.

Swim

"One minute to start," the announcer said. I felt strangely calm. I repeated to myself: *This is just a workout. Just a workout. This is just a long workout.*

The announcer boomed, "Thirty seconds to start." I counted down the seconds in my head. I said a quick prayer. As I said *Amen*, the starting gun went off and I pushed forward. Once my face hit the water, I was calm. I felt in control. I felt so strong. *Yes*, I thought, *this is going to be awesome!*

Then, I realized that I was experiencing the longest, saltiest swim in the history of the world. I had never seen so many buoys in my life. Yellow, red, orange. Hundreds of them. (Okay, maybe ten.) I pushed on, spitting sea grass out of my mouth. Ahead, I saw some pink swim caps, meaning that I had caught up to the previous wave. Forward progress!

More sea grass attacked me. And so did the men in the green cap and purple cap waves behind me. One guy swam over me. Literally. I felt a hand on my butt, then I felt an entire body go over me. Out of the corner of my eye, I saw a furry belly pass right over my face—and not in a sexy way. In an *OMG, I'm being killed* kind of way. Repeatedly, I was knocked around and kicked in the head. I was elbowed.

No matter how far to the side I attempted to be, to stay out of the way of the fast people, I was constantly in someone's way. At the same time, people were in *my* way, too. Maybe that's just open water swimming. We are fish without the ability to swim like fish and know our territory.

I rounded the last turn buoy and swam the last 500 meters to safety.

I walked my jelly legs up the stairs, and went through the fresh water rinse. As I "ran" to transition, I swore the crowd of people was judging me. I might as well have been naked. I felt huge and seriously out of place.

In that moment, I had a decision to make. Was I going to spend the entire race looking down? Thinking I did not belong? And why? Because

continues

continued

(to quote Bridget Jones): "I can't ski, I can't ride, I can't speak Latin, my legs only come up to here and yes . . . I will always be just a little bit fat"?

No. I was not going to do that. I had worked too hard. I held my salty head up, and made it alive into transition.

I had a good, rather uneventful T1, considering the distance to travel from the swim finish to the transition area. Gerry had mentioned how imprecise the fine motor skills can be in transition, which is part of the reason to practice transitions. This swim was the longest race swim I had done, and I noticed how correct he was. My fingers seemed to go in opposite directions.

Bike

The bike leg was ridiculous with its headwinds, side winds, rain, bumpy pavement, traffic, and railroad crossings. The ride was on a major roadway, and although the entire left lane was blocked off with orange cones for the race, the traffic was sketchy and scary. Coupled with horrendous winds, it was a nasty bike leg. I could not believe the amount of sheer cyclist carnage on the road. I saw a pileup of six superfit athletes on the side of the road heading out on the course and I was shaken to my core.

The bike was mostly this: "On your left" "On your left" "On your left" "On your left" "On your left" "On your left" "On your left" "On your left" "On your left" "On your left" "On your left" "On your left" "On your left" "On your left" "On your left!!!!"

Despite the headwind, I had a good time on the bike, averaging about 16.5 mph. The first half of the bike was much better, as the wind caught me hard core after the turnaround. I found plenty of time to be grateful during the bike portion, despite the evil winds and tough conditions. I spent moments thanking God for the day, and I really took the time to appreciate that I was halfway through the race—and still alive.

On the left, experienced cyclists blew by. On the right, eighteen-wheeler trucks blew by.

I hit the bike wall about Mile 44. I wanted off that bike. The Queen was an angry, bitter Queen at this point. I stood up in the saddle to give her some relief, but she yelled louder when I sat back down. I decided she would have to tough it out. So, the Queen was angry, and I was

continues

continued

also hungry, but sort of shaky and not feeling like swallowing anything. I did take a few salt tabs, because the sun had come out, promising a hot run.

I had never been so glad to see a sign in my life: BIKE IN. After an uneventful dismount (thank you, sweet Lord), I limped to my transition spot.

Run

I ran out of transition, feeling pretty good. *Run and done, run and done*, I repeated to myself, over and over. I had a two-loop course ahead of me. As I've mentioned, I like two-loop courses almost as much as I like childbirth. I started off pacing at about a 12:00-minute mile, which according to my training, would have been reasonable. Strategically, I was thinking, I could finish with about a 12:30 pace.

At the Mile 1 sign, I almost cursed out loud. Mile 1? Mile 1?! *That means I have 12.1 to go. 12.1! 12.1!*

My legs stopped working shortly thereafter. The legs were moving forward, but my hamstrings were not *firing*. I could not get the legs to *turn over*. Instead, I was dragging them behind me like tree trunks. By Mile 2, I knew I was in for a 70.3 special treat.

The run went over the McArthur Causeway, which on fresh legs would have been tough, although arguably fun. But after four hours of swimming and biking, the trek over the causeways did not bring "fun" to mind. I was thinking more along the lines of alien autopsy, or anal probe.

I jogged the first 3 miles of the run. I looked at my Garmin at one point, and I was chugging along at a 4.4 mph pace. *I can walk faster than this*, I thought. At the top of the bridge, I had to walk. I walked because I knew I had 9.5 miles to go. I trotted downhill, thinking that the turnaround was close, thinking that I could say I was one quarter complete. But I was wrong.

On the way back up the causeway, I started to feel a tad better. I had a few gels. Plus, the aid stations were awesome. With ice, water, Coke, bananas, oranges, there was something for me at every turn. I never thought I would want fruit during a race, but I devoured oranges at every turn. The texture was divine. After five solid hours of baby food (gels), real fruit was delicious.

continues

continued

However, I only felt good for a little while. I was beginning to cramp up a little, and my legs refused to turn over.

The first loop was bad. The second loop was hell.

As I headed down the home chute (but to start my second loop), the crowd was cheering. The spectators clearly thought I was about to finish. As I made the turn around, I was deflated. Another 0.2 virtually felt impossible. I walked for a solid five minutes, slowly moving right past the crowd that cheered me in.

The sun was out and the rain had stopped completely. The heat began to take over, wear me down. Somewhere on the way out on the second loop, I saw the Expert. I began to cry. I saw him coming for about 100 yards. The closer he got, the more I cried. We crossed, slapped hands, and he asked, "Are you okay?"

I sobbed, "Yes. I am just glad to see you. How do you feel?"

"Great!" he said.

Going up the causeway for the second time, I was wrecked. The left lane was blocked off for the runners, but traffic continued to flow in the right lane. Frankly, I was pretty disoriented. At one point, I lost my whereabouts, and I stumbled. A Mazda honked at me. I was over the cones, and I had no clue.

On and on I ran. I walked. I had *zero* grateful moments. Not because I wasn't grateful, but because I was lost. I was wandering. I do not remember much from Mile 7 to Mile 10. I just remember constantly talking to myself. With every footstep, I thought, *Just. Move. Forward. Just. Move. Forward. Just. Move. Forward.*

Bridge up, bridge down, bridge up, bridge down.

At Mile 8.5, I stopped to pee in a Porta-Potty. I opened the door, shut the door, locked the door. I turned around, and as my eyes adjusted to the darkness, I saw something on the seat. *What is that?* I wondered. I squinted. *Oh. That's poop. Poop. Poop. Poop.* I repeated it in my mind. "Crap," I said out loud.

Indeed.

I was in a Porta-Potty. I had been moving for going on six hours. I was tired. I was thirsty. I was hungry. And now, I was talking with a poo pile. I closed my eyes. And I hovered over it. *This is it*, I thought. *I am in this*

continues

continued

to finish, and finish strong. Because otherwise I truly cannot justify this moment. Poop. I cannot tell my kids one day that I peed, hovering over a stranger's poop, and then say, yeah, well I didn't finish that race. *Oh, hell no. I am going to finish.*

I kept moving. *Just. Move. Forward. Just. Move. Forward.* It was then I saw the Mile 9 sign. Four more miles. Four More. Miles. No. No. No.

With 1.5 miles to go, I saw a race volunteer. He was a long-haired, teenager—a kid, really. As I shuffled by him, behind my sunglasses with only a short distance remaining to completing my ultimate quest, he snickered, snorted, and then laughed at me.

I thought I was mistaken. But then he looked at me, nudged his buddy standing next to him, *pointed at me*, and snorted again.

I stopped.

For just a second. I stood still. I looked at him, and I said, "Did you @#%*ing just laugh at me?"

His little baby eyes grew big, and he turned away, embarrassed. I knew I had not imagined the scoffing when a crowd member said, "*YEAH!* What she said! Go, girl!"

Oh boy. A mean teenager laughed at me. What was I? A five-year-old? At this stage of the race? Yes. Yes, I was.

I kept going. *Just. Move. Forward. Just. Move. Forward.* Mile 12.5.

Before I knew it, I could hear the finish line. *Hear* the finish line? Yes.

Anyone who races knows exactly what I mean. Sometimes you can hear music, an announcer, and maybe some cheers. But somehow, I swear my ears ingest sounds of finish, applause, and satisfaction a few seconds before the ears could possibly physically, actually *hear* these sounds. Maybe it's the sheer *hope* for the finish that makes me hear things.

As I was running down the chute, I looked at my watch. I had hoped for a 6:50:00 time. I looked at my watch—7:14:00—and I was thrilled. I had made it. I took a few minutes to enjoy the run home. People clapped and cheered. I saw surprised faces, encouragement, laughter, smiles, and heard lots of "Go girl" and "Way to go!" I heard it all. When I saw the IRONMAN 70.3 Miami FINISH LINE banner, I put my hand on my heart, then my head, and I said, "Thank you, God. Thank you." And I meant it with every fiber of my being.

continues

continued

As I crossed the finish line, I threw out my thumbs-up, I did a fist pump, and I jumped. I was foolish.

It. Was. Done. I had finished 70.3 miles.

The Expert finished a little while later and I cried. Yes, again. I smelled like the dirtiest, smelliest billy goat in the entire world. Salt was crystallized on every surface of my skin. I was sunburned. I looked beaten. We had planned for a big night out. I had brought a fancy dress to wear. But we couldn't walk. We didn't want to walk. I could not hold my arms up to dry my hair. We decided the hotel restaurant was perfect. We devoured everything they had on the menu.

As I was stuffing cake into my mouth, Gerry called me.

"How is my finisher?" he asked.

"Hungry!" I said.

"What happened on your swim?" he asked.

"What do you mean?"

"Well, it was slow," he said, teasing me.

I said, "No, my run was slow!"

He laughed and turned on his serious voice, "Congratulations. I am so proud of you. You did the work. You earned your finish. Congratulations."

I got a little teary. "Thank you. For everything."

"Now," he said, "Tell me about the race. . . . "

THE GREAT TRIATHLON BEYOND

Whether you are embarking on your triathlon journey or continuing it, embrace this attitude of "I can and I will." Decide what you want, and decide that you *will*. This frame of mind is deliciously obnoxious, and will carry you far in your training and on race day.

People who are content to sit, to watch their lives roll on past, will not understand this kind of attitude. I was previously one of these people, but triathlon changed that perspective for me. When you find yourself on the grass-is-greener side of the motivational fence, be aware that others may not feel the love. Others may start to resent you for your new outlook on life. The resentment will start small and harmless, such as in the break room at work, "OMG, how can you get up at four thirty a.m. to go to the *gym*?" Then, the more determined you become, the more you will actually see the resentment, the eye-rolling, the snickers.

Even people close to you, people who love you may try to derail you. Say you will accomplish something big. Say it out loud, blog about it, scream it from the rooftops, and watch the negativity and resentment unfold right before your eyes. I watched it happen from the time St. Anthony's was a glimmer in my eyes until I crossed the finish line at several IRONMAN races. Actually, I still see it when I share my latest "exercise" adventures—whether it's triathlon or weightlifting competitions.

Outside negativity does one of two things *to* you when you are seeking to accomplish a new, scary goal:

1. It either thrusts you into "I'll show you" mode and acts as a facilitator for your training, or
2. It knocks you down completely, deflating your confidence and ending the goal.

Choose the first one. Stay focused. Let the bad days "go," and just do better the next day.

I hope you know how much *I* believe in you. I may have never met you, but here's what I accept as true: You can do a triathlon. You can do a sprint distance. You can do a half Ironman. You can do an Ironman. Just pick your poison—and go for it. You can do it. I believe in *you*, because I believed in myself—I could not swim, bike, or run worth a hill of beans two years ago—but with some hard work, I finished 70.3 miles. Then, I finished another. And then IRONMAN. And then another. And then I tackled more things, such as CrossFit and marathons, and on and on.

You can do this. So much joy, potential, and inspiration starts now. It's yours for the taking. *Carpe triathlon.*

REPEAT AFTER ME

Whatever your goal, show the naysayers, the negative people and the haters who you are.

Better yet, prove yourself to yourself. You are the one who matters.

Let the only person who can stop you . . . be you.

Believe in yourself.

You are stronger than you imagine.

Tell yourself: "Yes. I. Can. And. I. Will."

Take one step, one day, one hour at a time.

But always . . .

Just keep moving forward, my friend.

APPENDIX A

HOW TO SPEAK TRIATHLON

25-meter pool—64 lengths equal 1 mile.

25-yard pool—70 lengths equal 1 mile.

400-meter track—A track that is regulation will be 400 meters for one lap; four times around will equal 1 mile.

Aerobic—Exercise that easy on your system, allowing body to train with oxygen and delivering such to the muscles. See "Go Slow to Go Fast," page 134.

Aero—Term to describe the "aerodynamic" position of an athlete on the bike or also the swim.

Age group/age grouper—Divisions in triathlon races. Usually, the divisions are divided into gender and age; for example, Female 35–40. There are other optional divisions, such as "Athena" and "Clydesdales."

Anaerobic—Exercising at a pace/intensity that builds lactic acid quickly—because your respiratory and cardiovascular systems cannot deliver all or most of the oxygen required by your muscles. The pace associated with anaerobic running cannot be sustained very long. Example: the 40-yard dash.

Anaerobic threshold (AT)—Also known as lactate threshold; the transitory place between aerobic and anaerobic running. Training will allow your muscles to use oxygen more efficiently, so that less lactic acid is produced.

AquaBike—A race that leaves out the run. Swim and bike only.

Athena Division—An *optional* female division to enter in *some* races. Instead of entering into the age group, a female can choose "Athena," which is women who are 165 pounds or higher.

Body marking—In a race, you will be required to wear your race number on your body, often on the upper arm, lower leg, or sometimes the thigh. Before a race, there will be designated "body markers," volunteers who write your race number on your body with either a permanent marker, or applying a temporary peel-off tattoo.

Bonk—Also known as "hitting the wall." The point where you feel that you cannot go another step due to the glycogen in your muscles being overly depleted.

Bottle cage—The rack installed on your bike to hold your water bottle.

Cadence—Also known as revolutions per minute (rpm), *cadence* means the rhythm of your swim stroke, bike pedal stroke, or run turnover of the feet (as they hit the ground), which is usually measured in rpms.

Check-in—Before a larger race, the race may require you to check yourself and/or your bike in. Read the rules of each race carefully so you will know.

Cleat—The part on the bottom of the cycling shoe where your shoe attaches to your clipless pedals.

Clipless pedals—Pedals installed on your bike that allow you to "clip in" your shoes. These help your feet remain attached to the bike so you can use a full revolution in your pedaling.

Clydesdale—The boy version of the Athenas—male racers weighing over 220 pounds.

CO_2 cartridge—Sold at bike stores, these are essentials for your bike bag for inflating a tube with a touch of a button.

Derailleur—A system on a mountain bike, road bike, or triathlon bike, made of up sprockets and a chain with a method to move the chain from one to the other—this causes the shifting of gears.

DNF—Acronym for "Did Not Finish" (the race).

DNS—Acronym for "Did Not Start" (the race).

Drafting—Most commonly a term used in cycling, drafting entails riding close behind the rider ahead of you to avoid wind drag and assist in decreasing your effort.

Duathlon—A race consisting of run and bike and run again.

Fartlek—Another name for interval training that creates a mix of recovery-pace running, moderate pace, and short, fast bursts. Fartlek training is a fun and possibly silly way to increase speed and endurance. The word itself is fun.

Foam roller—A training tool (torture device) made out of cylindrical stiff foam that helps release "trigger points" in your muscles as you roll your body across them.

Foot strike—How your foot makes contact with the ground when walking or running. Jury is (still) out on which is best.

Gels—A form of sports nutrition typically used by triathletes in races due to the ease of digestibility, quick energy, and convenience.

Goggles—Protective eyewear for the swim, not to be confused with "Googles."

Half IRONMAN 70.3 distance—a triathlon event consisting of a 1.2-mile swim, a 56-mile bike, and a 13.1-mile half marathon run (total of 70.3 miles). Note that "IRONMAN" is a registered trademark of the World Triathlon Corporation and while some races may consist of the "half Ironman" distance of 70.3 miles, there is only one official IRONMAN 70.3 brand.

Half marathon—A race consisting of a 13.1-mile run.

Hill repeats—Just as it sounds. Running or riding up hills and down hills, and then turning around and doing it again. For as many times as required by training plan, coach, or insanity.

Holding the line—Imagine when you are pedaling on your bike that you are following a solid line. Holding your line is necessary for group rides and general bike safety.

Indoor trainer—A contraption that allows you to ride your bike indoors, essentially transforming it into a stationary bike.

Intervals—Training using short, fast "repeats" or "repetitions." Interval training builds speed and endurance. Another term for "pure misery."

IRONMAN—A branded triathlon event consisting of a 2.4-mile swim, a 112-mile bike, and a 26.2-mile marathon run (total of 140.6 miles).

IT band—The iliotibial band, which is a band of tissue that runs along the outside of the thigh, over the hip, down the knee, and below the knee. The IT band keeps the knee stable during walking and running.

Kickboard—A flat rectangular piece of Styrofoam used to isolate leg muscles in kick sets.

Lactate threshold—See "Anaerobic threshold."

Lane— Place in the pool where a swimmer swims; if you pick a lane, by all means, stay in it. Learn how to share.

Lap—Distance from one end of the pool to the other end . . . and back.

Length—Distance from one end of the pool to the other.

Long course triathlon—Typically considered anything over an Olympic distance race. Also, see "IRONMAN" and "IRONMAN 70.3."

Lube—Can be used to keep your chain on your bike greased; other types of lube include Aquaphor, BodyGlide, and Hoo Ha Ride Glide, and those lubes can be used under your arms, under the bra strap(s), between the knees, and anywhere else you might experience chafing. On the bike, make sure you lube your chain . . . and the Queen.

Marathon—A running race consisting of 26.2 miles.

Mash—To push a higher (heavier/harder) gear while riding on a bike. Usually, *mashing* means slowing your cadence and really pushing the bike pedals hard. Typically, "mashers" are at a disadvantage in cycling, as you are really looking to have optimization between power and cadence. When you are mashing, you aren't maintaining an efficient cadence that can go the distance.

Mini-Sprint—Shorter than a Sprint Distance triathlon. Usually a great beginner distance that can include a swim as short as 300 meters, a bike around 8 miles, or a run less than a 5K.

Mountain bike—A bike designed to be used off-road; that is, on such surfaces as trails and in the woods.

Off-Road Triathlon—Usually a swim, mountain bike, and trail run race, as opposed to a swim, road bike, and road run race.

Olympic Distance—May also be known as an "Intermediate Distance" or a "Short Course Triathlon" and usually a race of a 0.9-mile swim, 26-mile bike, and 10K (6.2-mile run).

"On Your Left"—The safety phrase to alert someone *on your right* that you are coming up *on the left* and passing . . . *on the left*.

Overpronation—Excessive inward rolling of the feet during running or walking.

Paddles—These make you look like a frog in the water and are worn on your hands to help build your stroke strength.

Plank—An abdominal exercise used for strengthening the core of the body. Looks like the start of a push-up position, only resting on forearms and elbows, and holding the position for periods of time; builds endurance in the abdominals and back, as well as the core stabilizer muscles.

PB—Acronym for "personal best."

PR—Acronym for "personal record."

Pull float—A floatation device used between the knees while swimming, which aids in keeping the bottom half of your body up in the water and allowing you to concentrate on your stroke.

Puncture—A flat tube.

Queen—Meredith Atwood lingo for your bottom-half lady parts.

Race belt—A belt where you can attach your race number and if you are lucky, hide snacks. This is helpful for putting on your number after the swim. You clip the belt around your waist with your number to the back (on the bike—if required by the race), and then when you run, you rotate your number to the front. You do *not* swim in your race number.

Rim—On a bike, the rim is the outside of the bike wheel that holds the tire in place.

Road bike—A bike made for traveling on paved roads; they are lighter than cruising or mountain bikes and have many gears with which to confuse you. Typically, the road bike will have the skinny, high-pressurized tires for a smoother ride.

Road rash—A slang term for the scrapes and abrasions resulting from your sweet lady skin hitting the hard, evil pavement.

RPM—See "Cadence."

Saddle sores—Ride too far, too early, and without lube and your rear end will learn about these.

Spinning—To pedal at a relatively easy, but high cadence; also, short for indoor cycling classes. However, note that Spin, Spinner, Spinning, and the Spinning logo are all registered trademarks owned by Mad Dogg Athletics, Inc.

Split—Typically used to describe the time it takes you to do a sport in the race. For example, the "bike split" would be your time from the start of the bike portion of the race, to the time you enter T2.

Sprint triathlon—A short distance triathlon usually consisting of approximately a quarter-mile swim, 15-mile bike ride, and 5K (3.1-mile) run. Distances vary, but they are on the "short" side.

Strike—See "Foot strike."

Swim sets—The way a swim workout is written.

Swim wave—Most races divide the start of the event into "waves." That means that groups start at different times, thus keeping the crowding on the swim down, but also on the entire course. In larger longer-distances races, such as Ironman races, sometimes there is only one swim wave.

T1—See "Transition."

T2—See "Transition."

Taper—The period of time before a race where you slow down the frequency and intensity of the workouts to give your body time to recover and rest before the event. The taper will make you crazy.

Timing chip—Usually handed out in race packets, these may be worn on your shoes (running race) or on an ankle strap (triathlon). When you pass over certain points during a race, the timing chip registers your time for the official race results.

Tire lever—Small plastic tool for your bike bag. The tire lever helps you remove the flat tire tube from the rim of the wheel.

Toe clips—The in-between of regular bike pedals and clipless pedals. You can ride your bike with sneakers and clip your toes into these plastic clips installed on your pedals to give you the benefit of a full revolution on the bike without the beginner scariness of clipless pedals.

Trainer—See "Indoor trainer."

Transition—Two time periods within a triathlon. T1 is the period of time between the swim and bike; T2 is the period of time between the bike and the run. See Chapter 14.

Triathlete—One who competes in a triathlon, also known as *you.*

Triathlon bike—A type of road bike that is specifically and ergonomically designed to keep the rider in a more streamlined and aerodynamic position. See Chapter 7.

Tri kit—A matching top and bottom often worn during a race. The material is meant to wear from start to finish, during the swim, bike, and run, and if necessary, under the wetsuit.

Tube—On a bike, the tube is the inflatable part *inside* the tire. You remove the tube, not the tire, when you have a flat.

Wave—See "Swim wave."

USAT—USA Triathlon (USAT) is the sanctioning authority for triathlon. You will likely need to join or buy a day pass to race in most events. Learn more at www.usatriathlon.org.

Wetsuit—A neoprene suit worn during open water swim training and races. The neoprene suit is to protect against cold water, but also to provide buoyancy.

Wicking material—A poly-blend fabric that does not absorb sweat (as cotton does), but instead shifts moisture away from the skin.

APPENDIX B

YOUR TRAINING PLAN

THIS TRAINING PLAN IS MAPPED OUT BASED ON YOUR *CURRENT* experience level. Just answer the following simple questions to gauge which plan to use. Once you have your plan level, then you are good to start training with the plan.

GETTING STARTED: A QUIZ!

QUESTION 1: HOW FAR CAN I SWIM—RIGHT NOW?

A. I can't swim. At all.
B. I know *how*, but it's tragic looking and I feel like drowning. Maybe 3–4 laps. Total.
C. I'm a good or great swimmer.

QUESTION 2: HOW LONG CAN I BIKE—RIGHT NOW?

A. What's a bike?
B. 10 to 20 minutes.
C. 30 minutes or more.

QUESTION 3: HOW FAR CAN I RUN—RIGHT NOW?

A. I do not run or jog. I walk.

B. Up to 2 miles.

C. I could complete a 5K or more.

If you are mostly A's, then go with the True Beginner Plan. Mostly B's? Try the Beginner Plan. Mostly C's? Then, head on to the Three-Month Plan. Feel free to mix and match as the sports require. For example, if you are a proficient swimmer but a newbie runner and cyclist, then jump right into the Three-Month Plan for the swim, and pick up on the Beginner or True Beginner Plan for the bike or run.

TRUE BEGINNER PLAN

Much like its name, the True Beginner Plan is for someone who is completely new to triathlon. Heck, this plan is for someone completely new to *exercise* or *movement* other than from the couch to work.

For example, when I started out with my first race, I was definitely a True Beginner. I had no idea what triathlon meant, how to properly run or ride my bike without falling. I could only sputter down one lane of a pool.

The True Beginner Plan will give you a jumping-off point to learn about triathlon and get moving in the right direction.

Time: Cross the finish line of your first race in nine months.

BEGINNER PLAN

The Beginner Plan is for someone who has dabbled in swimming, biking, or running, and who is able to handle small amounts of activity right now. You are not straight off the couch, but you aren't qualifying for the Olympics, either. I like to think of this category as the classic gym-goer who is ready to do tri.

Time: First race within 6 months of starting.

THREE-MONTH PLAN

The Three-Month Plan is for someone who can swim, bike, and run well, but has never put together all three into a triathlon. As the name allows, you will cross the Finish line in three months.

USING THE TRAINING PLAN

Use your answers in the Training Checklist to decide whether you fall under the True Beginner, Beginner, or Three-Month Plan.

Feel free to mix and match the plans depending on your skill level. For example, if you are beginning as a swimmer and cyclist, but are an avid runner, just go with the Three-Month Run Plan for the run, but use the True Beginner Plan for the swim and bike.

If in doubt and you are completely new to exercise or sport, go with the True Beginner Plan.

TRUE BEGINNER PLAN
9 Months to Race Day

The idea behind the beginner plan is to start training for your first tri in the "season." Typically, the triathlon "season" starts in April or so, depending on where you live. So, back out the nine months that is required by this plan and see where your first triathlon can be, time-wise. Again, this is a broad structure—if you want to try seven months, go ahead! Don't be held captive by any training plan. At the same time, make sure that you are prepared for race day.

DAYS YOU WILL WORK OUT

	Sunday	Monday	Tuesday	Wednesday	Thursday	Friday	Saturday
Swim			X		X		
Bike				X			X
Run	X			X*		X	
Core / Strength	X					X	

*After Month 6, only do you add the run after the bike for the "Brick" workout.

TRUE BEGINNER PLAN: SWIM

TIME FRAME: 9 MONTHS

If you have no earthly idea how to swim the freestyle stroke, the first step is learning the basics of this stroke. I recommend three to six swim lessons to get you started. Once you can reasonably swim one or two pool lengths, begin working on your regular swim plan, as follows.

DAYS TO SWIM:

Tuesdays, Thursdays

STARTING OUT:

After you feel comfortable enough with swimming a length of the pool without stopping and after your lessons are complete, then you are ready to begin the training program. To start for the first few weeks, aim only to swim 200 to 400 yards/meters each session (8 to 16 lengths of the pool). Yes, this may be hard. But in the swim, you will see the largest gains. Just keep swimming forward.

THE LINGO:

As you get more comfortable in the water, look online for swim "sets" that will help you find workouts that will break up the swim into sets. *Kick* means to use the kickboard and practice kicking down the pool. Most gyms with pools have kickboards for your use—just ask.

Swim means to freestyle swim.

Sets are written in shorthand like this: 2 x 100, 4 x 50. For the foregoing, it would mean to swim two sets of 100 meters with a rest in between. Then, swim four sets of 50 meters, with a rest in between each set.

A good example of a swim workout with sets (and the translation):

SAMPLE SWIM SET:

Warm-up: 100 meters, easy swim (*Translation:* use freestyle stroke unless otherwise designated)

Kick: 2 x 50 (*Translation:* you swim two sets of 50 meters with the kickboard while kicking your feet)

Main Workout: 2 x 100 w/:30 btw (*Translation:* swim 100 meters freestyle, rest 30 seconds "between," then repeat);

3 x 50:10 btw (*Translation:* swim 50 meters, rest 10 seconds, then repeat 2 more times for a total of 3);

100 pull (*Translation:* swim 100 meters with a pull float between your knees);

2 x 50—25 easy, 25 hard (*Translation:* just as it says, go slow down the length of the pool, then swim hard back—do this 2 times);

3 x 50, descend (*Translation:* go faster each set of 50 meters— you do this 3 times)

Cooldown: 100 easy

SAMPLE WORKOUTS:

Month 1:
  GOAL: Swim 200 to 500 meters each workout in Month 1
  Warm-up Kick: 50 meters
  Example Main Set: 4 x 50:30 btw; 100; 4 x 50 (25 easy, 25 hard)
  Cooldown

Month 2:
  GOAL: Swim 400 to 600 meters each workout
  Warm-up
  Kick: 50
  Example Main Set: 2 x 100:30 btw; 4 x 50 descend; 4 x 25 (25 easy, 25 hard)
  Cooldown

Month 3:
  GOAL: Swim 600 to 700 meters each workout
  Warm-up
  Kick: 100
  Drill: 100
  Drill Set: 25 fingertip drag drill, swim, 25 fist, swim
  Main Set: 100; 4 x 50 descend; 50 + 100 + 200:15 btw; 2 x 50
  Cooldown

Month 4:
  GOAL: Swim 700 to 800 meters each workout
  Warm-up
  Kick: 100
  Drill: 100

Drill Set: 25 fingertip drag drill, swim, 25 superman, swim

Main Set: 4 x 50 descend; 100 pull; 200 hard; 4 x 50 (25 easy, 25 hard); 100 Cooldown

Month 5:

GOAL: Swim 800 to 1,000 meters each workout

Warm-up

Kick: 100

Drill: 100

Drill Set: 25 fist, swim, 25 superman, swim

Main Set: 500-meter time trial continuous; 200 pull; 8 x 50:15 btw

Cooldown

Month 6:

GOAL: Swim 1,000 to 1,200 meters each workout

Warm-up

Kick: 100

Drill: 100

Main Set: 100 pull; 6 x 100 (50 easy, 50 hard)

100 continuous; 3 x 100:30 btw

Cooldown

Month 7:

GOAL: Swim 1,100 to 1,400 meters each workout

Warm-up

Kick: 100

Drill: 150

Main Set: 1,000-meter time trial; 8 x 50 (25 easy, 25 hard)

Cooldown

Month 8:

GOAL: Swim 1,200+ meters each workout

Warm-up

Kick: 150 to 200

Drill: 100 to 200

Main Set: 8 x 50; 50 + 100 + 200 + 400 + 200 + 100 + 50:30 btw; 100

Cooldown

Month 9:

GOAL: Swim 1,400+ meters each workout

Warm-up

Kick: 100 to 200

Drill: 150 to 200

Main Set: 400 (100 pull, 100 swim, 100 pull, 100 swim);
   8 x 50; 4 x 100

Cooldown

OPEN WATER:

Do *not* go into open water until Month 5, 6, or 7, or until you feel *very* comfortable in a pool. Just remember: never swim alone and learn your safety stroke.

TRUE BEGINNER PLAN: BIKE

DAYS TO BIKE:

Wednesday, Saturday

DISTANCE:

On Wednesday, take a spinning class at your gym, if available. This will help prepare your cycling muscles, the Queen, and your rear end.

On Saturday, venture out and take your bike for a ride in a safe place if you can for your "long ride." The following distances are goals for mileage for your long ride. Stay away from heavily trafficked areas until you know the rules of the road and are comfortable on your bike. Alternatively, you can go off time only—starting with fifteen to thirty minutes and working up to over two hours by the end of Month 9 for your long ride.

Month 1:

3 to 8 miles per ride

Month 2:

5 to 10 miles

Month 3:

7 to 12 miles

Month 4:

9 to 15 miles

Month 5:

12 to 18 miles

Month 6:

15 to 20 miles

Month 7:

18 to 22 miles

Month 8:

21 to 25 miles

Month 9:

25 to 28 miles

Remember to learn the rules of the road. Stay alert at all times. Pay attention . . . and remember to enjoy yourself!

TRUE BEGINNER PLAN: RUN

The goal with run is to get your *time* in—meaning that you need to do the *amount* of time on the clock to build your endurance base and work up to longer distances. Do *not* worry about how far you go in the beginning. If you must walk, then walk. Jog where you can, but get the mileage in. See the Run Section, page 133, regarding heart rate training. The Zone 2 runs would be your "jog"—so use easy and conversational paces. The hills and intervals, however, would be a little more breathy with a higher heart rate.

DAYS TO RUN:

Sunday, Wednesday (only for "Bricks" and after Month 4; and Friday

DISTANCE:

Just keep moving for the allocated time in the plan. By the time you get to Month 9, you will be jogging 3 to 5 miles (or more!) easily. Remember to check out the Galloway Method (www.GallowayMethod.com) for run-walk intervals.

Do not be captive to this plan. You can go further and longer, or jump ahead if you find it's too easy. Stay at a distance/time for an extra few weeks if you are feeling that you are too tired or the time is too long. Adjust as needed. Be careful to listen to your body and your soul. Your body will tell you its limits—and you *should* push its limits sometimes. But listen to your pain limits. Listen to your soul. If you feel bad or are sick one day, lay off.

Month 1:
   15-minute walk/jog per workout

Month 2:
   30-minute walk/jog

Month 3:
   35-minute walk/jog

Month 4:
   40-minute walk/jog

Month 5:
   40-minute walk/jog

Month 6:
   30- to 40-minute jog (add intervals and hills once a week)

Month 7:
   35- to 45-minute jog (add intervals and hills once a week)

Month 8:
   40- to 50-minute jog (add intervals and hills once a week, in a shorter run)

*Month 9:
   50- to 60-minute jog (add intervals and hills once a week, in a shorter run)

*The week before the race, slow down and "taper." This means to stretch, cycle, and run short(er) distances with easy effort. You want to be rested for race day.

Method

You will have about two or three run workouts per week. After a few weeks or months (depending on your progress), you will want to incorporate speed work (or track workouts), hill running, and longer, slower runs during these runs. As you get more comfortable, you can devote entire runs to hills, or speed. But integrate a little speed, hills, and lower–heart rate runs each week.

Brick

After Month 6, add an *additional* run workout to a cycling day *twice* a month. Ride your allotted time for your cycling workout, then add ten to twenty minutes of jogging immediately after the ride—the "brick" workout.

Core

Core workout on two run days: crunches, leg raises, and learn to plank. Incorporate some body-weight stability work and strength as well: lunges, body-weight squats, and hip and glute work, such as bridges.

Recovery

Monday is your Fun Day (off day) each week. Adjust as needed. Every fourth week should be a recovery week. This does not mean to take the week off and eat cookies—just dial back the distances and effort, and allow your body time to recover for the next cycle!

BEGINNER PLAN
Six Months to Race Day

DAYS YOU WILL WORK OUT

	Sunday	Monday	Tuesday	Wednesday	Thursday	Friday	Saturday
Swim			X			X	X*
Bike				X			X
Run	X				X		X*
Core / Strength				X		X	

*Alternate swim before run, and run after bike every other week *after* Month 3

BEGINNER PLAN: SWIM

TIME FRAME: 6 MONTHS

This is the plan if you know how to swim, but you are a bit of a flailer or perhaps need help with endurance. Get focused on your technique, so you feel more comfortable in the water. Concentrate on your stroke, your breathing and your form.

DAYS TO SWIM:

Tuesdays, Fridays.

Every other week after Month 3, add a long/open water swim before your bike ride.

STARTING OUT:

To start for the first few weeks, aim only to swim 200 to 400 yards/meters each session (8 to 16 lengths of the pool).

PLANNED DISTANCES:

See True Beginner Plan for lingo and explanations of swim sets.

Month 1:

GOAL: Swim 700 to 800 meters each workout

Warm-up

Kick: 100

Drill: 100

Drill Set: 25 fingertip drag drill, swim, 25 superman,
    swim

Main Set: 4 x 50 descend; 100 pull; 200 hard; 4 x 50
    (25 easy, 25 hard); 100 Cooldown

Month 2:

GOAL: Swim 800 to 1,000 meters each workout

Warm-up

Kick: 100

Drill: 100

Drill Set: 25 fist, swim, 25 superman, swim

Main Set: 500-meter time trial continuous; 200 pull;
    8 x 50:15 btw

Cooldown

Month 3:

GOAL: Swim 1,000 to 1,200 meters each workout

Warm-up

Kick: 100

Drill: 100

Main Set: 100 pull; 6 x 100 (50 easy, 50 hard)

100 continuous; 3 x 100:30 btw

Cooldown

Month 4:

GOAL: Swim 1,100 to 1,400 meters each workout

Warm-up

Kick: 100

Drill: 150

Main Set: 1,000-meter time trial; 8 x 50 (25 easy,
    25 hard)

Cooldown

Month 5:

GOAL: Swim 1,200+ meters each workout

Warm-up

Kick: 150 to 200
Drill: 100 to 200
Main Set: 8 x 50; 50 + 100 + 200 + 400 + 200 + 100 +
    50:30 btw; 100
Cooldown

Month 6:
GOAL: Swim 1,400+ meters each workout
Warm-up
Kick: 100 to 200
Drill: 150 to 200
Main Set: 400 (100 pull, 100 swim, 100 pull, 100 swim);
    8 x 50; 4 x 100
Cooldown

This may seem like a really long way to go in training for a
sprint triathlon, and yes, it is. However, you will feel prepared
and confident knowing you can swim this far before the race.

OPEN WATER:

Do not go into open water until Month 3 or 4 or until you feel
very comfortable in a pool. You may want to shoot for a pool
swim for your first triathlon if the water is an issue for you.
Swim at least three times in open water before your race
(preferably more). Learn to sight (keep your eye on the buoy
or other landmark) in order to stay on course.

BEGINNER PLAN: BIKE

DAYS TO BIKE:

Wednesday, Saturday.

DISTANCE:

On Wednesday, take a Spin class. Stay for an extra ten minutes after and ride a little longer after you've been training for
three months. On Saturday, hit the road with your bike and a
friend if you can.

Month 1:
   8 to 12 miles per ride

Month 2:
   13 to 15 miles

Month 3:
   15 to 18 miles

Month 4:
   18 to 22 miles

Month 5:
   22 to 25 miles

Month 6:
   25 to 30 miles

This may seem like a really long way to go in training for a sprint triathlon, and yes, it is. However, you will feel super-prepared and confident knowing you can ride 25+ miles in training to do a 10- to 15-mile ride in a race. Do it!

BEGINNER PLAN: RUN

Time to jog, baby. Start slowly and take time to learn proper mechanics. Have a running coach/trainer evaluate your run form as soon as you begin to *run*. Trust me—this is an injury saver. See the Run Section, page 133, regarding heart rate training. The Zone 2 runs would be your "jog"—so, easy and conversational paces. The hills and intervals, however, would be a little more breathy with a higher heart rate.

DAYS TO RUN:

Monday, Thursday, and Saturday (Add Brick workout after Month 3, once a week to your Saturday workout). Remember to check out the Galloway Method (www.GallowayMethod .com).

DISTANCE:

Month 1:
1-mile walk/jog per workout

Month 2:
1- to 2-mile jog

Month 3:
1.5- to 2.5-mile jog (add hills and intervals)

Month 4:
2.5- to 3-mile jog (add hills and intervals)

Month 5:
3- to 4-mile jog (add intervals and hills once a week, in a shorter run)

Month 6:
4- to 5-mile jog (add intervals and hills once a week, in a shorter run)

*The week before the race, slow down and "taper." This means to stretch, cycle and run short(er) distances with easy effort. You want to be rested for race day.

METHOD

You will have about three run workouts per week. You will want to incorporate speed work (or track workouts), hill running, and longer, slower runs during these runs. As you get more comfortable, you can devote entire runs to hills or speed. But integrate a little speed, hills, and lower–heart rate runs each week.

BRICK

After Months 2 through 3, add an *additional* run workout to a cycling day *twice* a month. Let Wednesday to be flexible. Ride your allotted time for your cycling workout, then add twenty to thirty minutes of jogging immediately after the ride, simulating race day.

CORE

Core workout on two run days: crunches, leg raises, and learn to plank. Add glute bridges, bodyweight squats, lunges, and upper body where available.

RECOVERY

Sunday is your Fun Day (off day) each week. Adjust as needed. Every fourth or fifth week should be a recovery week. This does not mean to take the week off and eat cookies—just dial back the distances and effort, and allow your body a time to recover for the next cycle.

THREE-MONTH PLAN

3 Months to Race Day

DAYS YOU WILL WORK OUT

	Sunday	Monday	Tuesday	Wednesday	Thursday	Friday	Saturday
Swim			X		X		X*
Bike				X**			X
Run	X			X**		X	
Core / Strength			X			X	

*Open Water Swim—see plan.
**Brick Workout—see plan.

THREE-MONTH PLAN: SWIM

You know how to swim, but you need to hone your skills.

DAYS TO SWIM:

Tuesday, Thursdays. Every other week, add a long/open water swim before your bike ride.

PLANNED DISTANCE:

Swim 1,600 to 2,200 meters each swim session, thirty to sixty minutes per session. Incorporate speed drills, kicks, drills and continuous swim practices. See online articles, YouTube, and Beginner Plan for ideas, and add distance.

EXAMPLE SWIM WORKOUTS:

Workout 1:

Warm-up: 100 easy
Kick: 100
Drills: 25 superman, 25 fist, 50 fingertip drag
Main Set: 100; 4 x 50 descending (getting faster each 50) 100 pull; 8 x 25 fast; 2 x 200:30 btw; 3 x 100:30 btw
Cooldown: 100 easy

Workout 2:

Warm-up: 100 easy
Kick: 100
Drills: 25 superman, 25 fist, 50 fingertip drag
Main Set: 100 + 200 + 300 + 400 + 300 + 200 + 100 w/:30 btw;
Cooldown: 100 easy

Workout 3:

Warm-up: 100 easy
Kick: 100
Drills: 25 superman, 25 fist, 50 fingertip drag
Main Set: 1,200 meters continuous for time (record your time); 4 x 100 easy
Cooldown: 100 easy

RECOMMEND:

This is the level where you want to join the master's swim class at your gym. Incorporate such drills as fist, catch, backstroke, and others. You might want to introduce the pull float and other swim toys with guidance and care.

OPEN WATER:

Take to the open water once a month when time allows. Practice sighting. Learn to feel über-comfortable in the water so that on race day you are flying, not fearing.

THREE-MONTH PLAN: **BIKE**

You can ride a bike and you are comfortable with the rules of the road. Now it's time to get stronger and faster.

DAYS TO BIKE:

Wednesday, Saturday. Add an extra day if you are feisty.

DISTANCE:

On Wednesday, take a Spin class if you can't get outside. Preferably, get outside. But if you can't ride, then get to Spin class early or stay for twenty to thirty minutes and ride a little longer. On Saturday, hit the road with your bike. Add some hill repeats and speed work starting Month 2, depending on the terrain of your race. Try and train on the course or like-course terrain. Work on drills (see Cycling section, page 97), and ride with speedy and competitive friends to get faster.

Month 1:
15 to 20 miles per ride

Month 2:
20 to 25 miles

Month 3:
25 to 35 miles

THREE-MONTH PLAN: **RUN**

Time to go longer and also get faster. Check out interval workouts and hill repeats for added toughness. Make sure you pay attention to heart rate training zones. Read online for more information.

DAYS TO RUN:

Sunday, Wednesday,* Friday

*Add Brick workout once a week.

DISTANCE:

Month 1:
2-mile run each long run workout (gradually building)
One day of 1 to 2 miles with intervals or hills

Month 2:
3- to 4-mile long run each week (gradually building)
One to two days of 2 to 3 miles intervals/hills

Month 3:
4- to 6-mile long run each week (gradually building)
One to two days of 2 to 3 miles of intervals or hills
Remember: The week before the race, slow down and taper.

METHOD

You have about three run workouts per week. You will want to incorporate speed work (or track workouts), hill running, and longer, slower runs. The long runs are key for building the endurance (these are "slower"—Zone 2 runs). The speed work and hills will serve you well on race day. So, remember to mix it up and include both!

BRICK

Add a run workout to a cycling day once a week, or more—if you are feeling great. Ride your allotted time for your cycling workout, then add 1 to 2 miles of jogging immediately after the ride, building up gradual progression until you feel ready to race!

CORE

Ab and core workouts on two run days, one on swim day. Add 1 to 2 workouts for strength: upper body (push-ups, etc.), and lower body (squats, lunges, bridges).

RECOVERY

Monday is your Fun Day (off day) each week. Adjust as needed. Theoretically, every fourth week should be a recovery week. Listen to your body and make sure that you are recovering properly. Recovery is a discipline.

NOTES

Notes to Chapter 1

1. Jayne Williams, *Slow Fat Triathlete: Live Your Athletic Dreams in the Body You Have Now* (Da Capo Press, 2004).

Notes to Chapter 7

1. https://www.trainingpeaks.com/blog/joe-friel-s-quick-guide-to-setting-zones/.
2. Ibid.
3. Gale Bernhardt, "Solutions for Numb Toes While Cycling," Active.com, http://www.active.com/cycling/Articles/Solutions-for-Numb-Toes-While-Cycling.htm.

Notes to Chapter 8

1. http://www.jeffgalloway.com/training/walk_breaks.html.
2. http://video.nytimes.com/video/2011/11/02/magazine/100000001149415/the-lost-secret-of-running.html.
3. https://www.runnersworld.com/training/g20862002/dynamic-warmup-stretches/.
4. http://www.activerelease.com.

Notes to Chapter 10

1. Joe Friel, *Your First Triathlon* (Boulder, CO: VeloPress, 2006).

2. http://www.cnn.com/2012/02/21/health/chrissie-wellington-triathlete-champion/index.html?hpt=hp_c2.

3. Ibid.

Notes to Chapter 12

1. Chris Carmichael and Jim Rutberg, *The Time-Crunched Triathlete: Race-Winning Fitness in 8 Hours a Week* (Boulder, CO: VeloPress, 2010).

Notes to Chapter 13

1. http://www.inc.com/magazine/201111/stop-feeling-like-a-big-fat-loser.html.

Notes to Chapter 15

1. Mike Reilly, Episode 46 of "The Same 24 Hours Podcast," www.Same24HoursPodcast.com.

ACKNOWLEDGMENTS

Mom and Dad—for years of love, support, and (Dad) teaching me to carry all the groceries from the car in one trip. Papooh—I love you. Mombow—I miss you. James Atwood III, CEO of the Atwood Corporation—thank you for supporting and loving me through another wild ride. James and Stella—I am so proud to be your mom. You're the most amazing children—like, ever. Matthew—you're a great lizard. Linda Hanson—for your support and inspiration. To the rest of my family thank you and love you all.

Gerry Halphen—forever gratitude. Ansley Sebring, Carrie Hanson, Brett Daniels, Karen Whitlock, Beth Morris—for your friendships. Julia Polloreno, Nicole DeBoom, Mike Reilly, Brent and Kyle Pease, Chrissie Wellington, Jeff Galloway, Scott Rigsby, Megan Melgaard, Dani Grabol, Rachel Joyce—for your support, friendships, and encouragement. Dr. Hamid Sadri—always, for "fixing" me more times than I can count. Robyn Weller and Susan Wintersteen—you two know why. Dina Griffin—for your true expertise and friendship. Todd Nixon—for your unwavering commitment and hard work. Curtis Henry—all the bikes and such. Roger Smith and Mary Sprague—for shaping me as a writer. Mary Hartman— for letting me see that this book was not only a possibility, but too close to ignore. Marissa Connors, Judy Newberry, and Tammy Williams—thank you for years of everything. Oprah—because, well, Oprah.

Bridget Quinn and Danielle Svetcov—for setting an unforeseeable chain of events in motion. Renée Sedliar—the BEE—for believing in this book and taking a chance on *me*.

Klean Athlete, Huma Gel, Quintana Roo, Zoca Gear—for believing in me and supporting the dream of Swim Bike Mom for years and years. IRONMAN and Lifetime Fitness.

Atlanta-area coffee shops—for superb office space and clean bathrooms. My athletes, readers, supporters, "fans," haters and trolls—I am thankful for each and every one of you—all for different reasons, but always gratitude. The Grateful Sobriety group—grounded, one day at a time. God—by your Grace I am saved and forgiven (forgiven a lot—and for that I am grateful).

INDEX